The Hearing Ear Dog

Understanding, Selecting, and Training Your Service Dog for Deaf and Hard-of-Hearing Alert Work

By R. A. Williams

ISBN: 9781072264460

Table of Contents

This book is dedicated to the hardworking professionals at Service Dogs of New Mexico and Duke City Dog Academy.

Chapter 1: Introduction

Congratulations on your decision to train a Hearing Ear Dog! I am confident that you will enjoy years of peace, security, and increased freedom because of the particular services your dog will provide to you.

I wrote this book because too many people who could potentially benefit from a Hearing Ear dog are not aware that they exist. In the summer of 2018, while on an extensive tour of the southern United States with Honeybits (my Hearing Ear dog), I encountered many other people with hearing loss, including a profoundly Deaf woman. All of them were aware of Seeing Eye dogs and similar service animals, and many had dogs as pets. But very few of them were aware that Hearing Ear dog training is available or that the specific type of assistive behavior provided by a Hearing Ear dog qualifies the dog as a legitimate service animal. This book is an attempt to spread the word.

My hearing loss began when I was quite young but did not become disabling until my forties. I'm learning American Sign Language (ASL) but am nowhere near fluent. One of the things I've done to help me stay employed and active is to train a Hearing Ear Dog: a five-pound Chihuahua named Honeybits.

Contrary to popular belief, you do not have to be profoundly Deaf to benefit from a Hearing Ear dog. If you're hard of hearing, you are already fully aware of the limitations of the available adaptive technology. You are also aware of the way hearing problems can isolate people socially. A dog trained to alert you to things in your environment that you cannot hear can literally save your life.

In September 2018, the Albuquerque chapter of the Hearing Loss Association of America invited me to share my story with them, to introduce Honeybits, and to help spread the word about Hearing Ear dogs. This book is a continuation of that effort.

This book begins by discussing disability and service animals in general. It describes the criteria necessary to qualify a service animal and to distinguish between a legitimate service dog and a "pet in a vest". It discusses some of the legal issues related to service animals, along with some of the issues Deaf and hard-of-hearing people face. The emphasis is primarily on the laws and processes in the United States, however Deaf rights in other nations do vary and I spend some time discussing them. With rights come responsibilities, so there's information about what you, as the owner of a Hearing Ear dog, must do to remain on the right side of the law.

This book will describe, in detail, what a Hearing Ear dog *does*. Although most pet owners have noticed that their dog responds to things in his or her environment, and although Hearing Ear dog training does begin by taking advantage of the dog's natural reactions, the behaviors displayed by a Hearing Ear dog go far beyond the animal's natural response.

There's some debate in the dog training community as to which animals are "best" for service work. More than one kind of service work exists, and because of the high demand for service animals some people can and do train their own. This book therefore discusses some of the requirements for Hearing Ear dog work. It discusses the training process, the specific techniques used to train service dogs, and some of the methodology.

From time to time, I will share a picture or anecdote featuring my own Hearing Ear Dog, a little Chihuahua named Honeybits who weighs about five pounds. I trained her under the supervision of Service Dogs of New Mexico and the Duke City Dog Academy. She passed her Public Access test in April of 2019 and is now a fully qualified service dog for the purposes of the Americans with Disabilities Act.

You Don't Have to Be Totally Deaf to Benefit

Many people believe that they "aren't disabled enough" to qualify for an assistance animal. This is partly because the need for service animals greatly exceeds the supply. Charities and agencies that match animals with handlers try to serve the people with the most severe disabilities first. Deafness and hearing loss are also frequently trivialized in popular culture and not considered "real" disabilities that affect

2

everything from education to driving. After a lifetime of absorbing this message, it's understandable why so many of us don't believe we are important enough to deserve help.

My hearing loss was evident even as a child, but it did not become severe until I was an adult. As of this writing I still have some hearing and can be helped with hearing aids. I don't have to lip read all the time and my hearing aids help amplify sounds in the speech range of frequencies. But even with my hearing aids there are some frequencies that are just plain gone. I'm physically incapable of hearing a knock at the door unless I'm standing less than an arm's length away. Since many people refuse to use the doorbell, more than once I've been surprised in my home by a family member who, having been given a key for emergency use, knocked politely and then entered when I did not answer. I've slept through hotel fire alarms—not once, but twice. I can still drive, and with my hearing aids in I'm capable of noticing a siren, but I can't tell what direction it's coming from. At work, I can still get by with hearing aids and lip reading, which is good because I'm still in my mid-forties and will need to work for several more years before I am eligible to retire. Unlike many people, I have the kind of job where hearing loss is not a deal-breaker. I can support myself financially and I even adopted a teenager. But the social aspects of hearing loss have hit me hard.

I live alone and have no family in town except a daughter and a niece. My daughter moved out when she became an adult, as most grown children do, and she has her own job and concerns. Neither she nor my niece is available to babysit me, and frankly since I'm not even fifty years old yet, I wouldn't care to be babysat. I'm losing my hearing, not my brain or my basic competency. My skills are still in high demand as an engineer, a writer, a math tutor, and a non-profit administrator. I've got no business retiring just yet and there's no reason I shouldn't continue being an asset to the community instead of a burden on its social safety net.

With help from Honeybits, I no longer sleep through fire alarms. I can drive safely even in unfamiliar places, and I don't miss a quiet knock at the door even when the dishwasher is running or I'm doing laundry. When I'm out and around, Honeybits points in the direction of oncoming sirens and informs me when a stranger is approaching or when something on the stove is boiling over. The cute things she does and the way she connects me to the rest of the outside world have been a great benefit because they provide an emotional lift and connection I would not otherwise have. Thanks to her, I should be able to continue to live independently until I qualify for a (dog-friendly) assisted living center. Meanwhile, I can continue to drive and to work.

Having Honeybits has made the difference between me being a contributing member of society and me being a burden either on the state or on some unfortunate family member.

My Story

As I mentioned earlier, my hearing problems began when I was quite young. As a toddler I had frequent ear infections, however since I apparently did not act like I was in pain the infections passed unnoticed for a long time. But the buildup of pus and fluid in my ears made it hard for me to hear. Eventually it reached the point when I could not hear my mother standing right behind me calling my name, at which point she realized I couldn't hear her and took me in for testing.

I ended up having my adenoids removed and tubes put in my ears when I was two. These worked, but my hearing was never good especially out of my left ear. I noticed it gradually deteriorating until, as an adult in my forties, I realized I was lip reading. Testing showed that I'd lost more than half of my hearing, and at age forty-three I needed to take some kind of action to allow myself to continue working.

I was always aware that service dogs existed, but was never really a "dog person" growing up. It may have been because I was bitten in the face by an Afghan hound when I was about eighteen months old. Although I do not remember the incident, there were others that were probably just as significant. A neighbor's miniature Dachshund chased me regularly, and until fourth grade the only way I could get to school was by walking by the poorly socialized German Shepherd. This dog, confined all day to a back yard, terrorized the children by lunging, snapping, and occasionally breaking down the gate. From time to time, a few of the fifth or sixth graders would tease the dog or let it loose to stalk the smallest and slowest among the first and second-graders. Since I couldn't see very well or run very quickly, the dog's group of targets naturally included me. I remember my mother calling the city animal control office more than once. Looking back, I now realize how lonely, neglected, and abused that poor dog must have been. But at the time, my fear drove out all other observations and thoughts that might have otherwise led to compassion.

As a child, I was terrified of dogs. When I visited my uncles, aunts, and cousins out on their farms, I stayed indoors with a book rather than face the large, rambunctious farm dogs that routinely jumped on people, chased cars, and barked. But when I reached the fourth grade I realized that dogs were a fact of life and that I'd have to do something to get rid of the fear.

I noticed that although a real dog could reduce me to a cowardly mess just by lunging and snapping at me, I could *read* about dogs without having the same reaction. I could look at pictures of dogs and even say the word "dog". Also, I learned in yoga and martial arts classes that there were things I could do to notice and keep track of my breathing and heart rate. I began a two-year process in which I learned as much as I could about dogs and how best to interact with them whole not freaking out. During this time, I watched other people interact with dogs and gradually crept closer and closer until I was able to pet and even hold a cute puppy named Blackie who belonged to one of my fifth-grade friends. Bigger dogs took a little bit longer. (I have since learned that a competent therapist could have gotten the work done in a couple weeks. It took me two years to reinvent that particular wheel.)

The final test came when, while doing some mandatory door-to-door fundraising for my elementary school, I arrived at the acreage of one of our neighbors. They weren't home, but their three Dobermans were. In fact, they were loose. The dogs, who had a reputation for aggression and who had supposedly once bitten an adult, came around the corner as I rang the doorbell. I was badly outnumbered, there was nothing nearby I could have used as an improvised weapon (I looked), the clipboard I carried was too small to be an effective shield, and the closest help was a quarter of a mile away even if someone was outside to hear me were I to scream. No divine being swept down from the sky to rescue me. I knew that the only way I would survive would be if I could control my reactions long enough to get back to the main road without triggering an attack. So I dropped my pulse rate, stayed calm, backed slowly away, and eventually made it out of the pack's territory without triggering an attack. From that point on I was never afraid of dogs in an out-of-control way although I doubted I would ever bond emotionally with one. Birds and cats, yes—just not dogs.

Many years later, I moved far away from my family to live and work in New Mexico. Some years after that, I adopted a teenager. During a particularly rough patch—not all adoptions go smoothly—my daughter requested a small dog as an emotional support animal. One of her bio-relatives had a surplus Chihuahua puppy, whom she gave to my daughter. The dog's name started out as "Buttercup" but turned into "Honey" and later "Honeybits" courtesy of the neighborhood children.

Things went well for a couple of weeks, at which point my daughter suddenly lost interest in the puppy. Since the woman who gave Honeybits to us wasn't answering her phone, the pup did the only thing she possibly could: she bonded with me instead, nuzzling her nose into my bad ear and being soft and wiggly.

"Well," I said resignedly to the two-pound puppy, "I'd like you a lot better if you were a kitten or a baby bird, but you can stay."

From that point, I provided all of Honeybits's care. She slept with me, I came home from work at lunch to feed her, and I taught her where to make potty and how not to bite hard on people's feet or fingers. Gradually, and almost unnoticeably, the dog started to ignore my daughter and focus on me. The turning point came when my daughter left home for the first time. The puppy transferred her attention to me. My hearing loss diagnosis a few months later was easier to take because of my furry little friend. In a matter of weeks, I'd fallen madly in love with Honeybits.

By the time my otosclerosis and hearing loss was diagnosed, it had already affected my work and travel. I noticed I was lip reading nearly all the time in meetings and struggling with telephone conversations. I've slept through fire alarms at two different hotels, and was having difficulty telling whether I'm being paged on an intercom. I'd already transferred out of a work assignment that required me to travel a lot, not solely because of the hearing loss, but I was very worried that in addition to losing my music and my martial arts, I was going to lose travel too. My world was closing in, not just because of my home life but because my work options were gradually falling away and I was far too young to retire. I needed to do *something*. Fast.

Honeybits, during that time, was the only light in my life. She was full of energy and didn't mind very well, so I took her to obedience classes and on walks. She took to the obedience training like a cat to a roll of hanging toilet paper. She wasn't yappy, and she seemed to want to be with me and to please me. I taught her to tell me who was at the door: my daughter, a stranger, a friend, or someone who was trying to break in. It was at that point that I thought: perhaps this little dog can help me compensate for my hearing loss. But it took a long time for me to find someone qualified to help me train her. I was reluctant to reach out, partly because hearing loss at my age is such an embarrassing thing and partly because I was well aware that the world is full of people with disabilities far more severe than mine.

At some level, I was afraid that someone would say: "What in the world are you thinking? Service dogs are for people with *real* disabilities." Here I was, with not just a job but a profession that allowed me to pay my bills and to afford to train a service dog out of pocket. My goal of remaining able to continue working, living independently, traveling, and enjoying the finer things in life even as my hearing deteriorated seemed small and insignificant.

I was having trouble thinking of my hearing loss as a disability, because I really didn't want to put that label on myself. Also, because Honeybits was already helping me out a lot at home, I thought that my desire to take her with me traveling was, well, selfish. We could, and did, take a long road trip up to Wyoming while staying solely in dog-friendly hotels. I didn't need help commuting in well-known areas such as while going to work or shopping for groceries, and like most people with hearing impairment I dislike restaurants and noisy environments. So was it necessary—vitally necessary—to have Honeybits trained as a service dog? And, would I be allowed to simply continue training her? Or would they make me get rid of her and replace her with some random retriever? *That* I obviously couldn't allow: no way was I going to give up the only creature in town who loved me.

In the fall, I made contact with Service Dogs of New Mexico (SDNM). "I have a dog," I wrote, "and I think that with some training she can do this work for me." Some discussion followed, along with a home inspection and a vet certification. When I showed off the year-old puppy's repertoire of tricks, and when little Honeybits earned her Canine Good Citizen title a few weeks later, the team concluded that if the tiny Chihuahua could do the work, the tiny Chihuahua could have the job, vest and all. Accordingly, little Honeybits began the next stage of her training. We worked with Lenae Fassler and Jen Hunt from the Duke City Dog Academy (DCDA), who showed me how to use the basic positive reinforcement tools such as a clicker to teach Honeybits new behaviors in as little as a couple hours.

These days, Honeybits is my little ride-or-die buddy. I appreciate her small size because when we travel by car she can alert me to the direction of an oncoming siren. She's a great little travel companion because she seldom whines or complains unless she has to go to the bathroom. She's interested in whatever activities or tours are available, she is alert and engaged, and she will go to bed and wake up when it's time to do so. She doesn't get carsick unless we're on a mountain road, and she doesn't throw tantrums because we have to wait for something or because we have to change our plans due to the weather. Most humans I know don't travel half as well.

So far, Honeybits has been to seventeen different states. In late 2018 we completed an eight-state road trip. People ask me whether I'm afraid to travel "alone", but I think it's a stupid question. I'm never alone. Dog is with me.

Terminology

Before we get too deeply into our subject I'd like to spell out what I mean by specific words.

A "**service dog**" (often abbreviated SD) is an animal specially trained to assist a person with a diagnosed disability, by performing specific trained tasks to compensate for that disability.

A "**disability**" is a documented physical, mental, or emotional limitation that has been diagnosed by a qualified doctor. It is significant enough to require adaptive technology or support so that the person with the disability can continue to function.

An "**emotional support animal**", not necessarily a dog, provides emotional support but does not perform specific trained tasks. Emotional support dogs (often abbreviated ESD) are not trained to operate in new or chaotic environments the way service dogs are trained.

A "**Hearing Ear dog**" is a dog trained to assist a Deaf or hard-of-hearing person by detecting important things in their environment and alerting that person by using a trained signal of some sort.

An "**alert dog**" is a dog trained to notify a handler of a specific thing or event in the handlers environment. Alert behavior can be a disability specific task.

A "**handler**" is the person who owns, walks, and "handles" the dog. In the case of a service dog, the handler is the person with a disability whom the dog is being trained to help. The handler participates in at least some of the training with the dog and frequently practices with the dog at home especially during the later stages of the animal's training.

A "**trainer**", who is generally *not* the handler, is a professional animal behavioral specialist. To work with service animals, a trainer generally possesses formal credentials from the American Kennel Club and other objective sources certifying his or her level of qualification. Not all animal trainers are qualified to administer the Public Access Test. Trainers who work with service dogs and their handlers are also familiar with different kinds of disabilities. Hearing Ear dog trainers are generally fluent in sign language because it allows them to communicate more effectively with the handler.

A "**task**" is a specific behavior or kind of work that is performed by a service dog to compensate for a handler's disability. Guide dogs for the blind steer their handlers around obstacles. Hearing Ear dogs alert their handlers to things in their environment they cannot otherwise hear. Medical alert dogs detect seizures, drops in blood sugar, and other medical problems in time for their handlers to react. Dogs can also perform bracing, fetching, operation of light switches, and other activities related to the handler's disability. It is legal for a business owner or employee to ask what tasks a service dog is trained to perform for the benefit of the handler.

The "**Canine Good Citizen**" (CGC) title is granted by the American Kennel Club when a dog—not necessarily a service dog—passes a test that is administered by an authorized and licensed trainer. This test evaluates whether the dog in question knows how to walk politely on a leash, sit and lie down on command, and perform basic obedience tasks.

"**Duke City Dog Academy**" (DCDA) is a business that provides dog training services to the public and to various businesses and government agencies. It's based out of Albuquerque, New Mexico. Other similar businesses exist all over the world, providing animal training that ranges from basic obedience to movie stunt work to, well, service animal training.

"**Service Dogs of New Mexico**" (SDNM) is a registered 501(c)(3) tax exempt charity that provides service dogs to people who need them. They provide education and orientation to prospective service dog handlers along with the screening, testing, and selection of prospective service dogs. Most of the actual training is subcontracted to professional trainers such as the ones who work for DCDA.

The "**Public Access Test**" is a rigorous test of a dog's ability to behave well in public. It contains none of the disability-specific trained behavior that is necessary for a dog to help a handler compensate for a disability. It focuses almost exclusively on safety, manners, and leash handling in a variety of situations. To pass the Public Access Test, a dog must get into and out of a vehicle, display correct parking lot safety and manners, and refrain from reacting to other people or dogs with aggression, fearfulness, or solicitations for play or attention. Not all states necessarily require service animals to pass a public access test, however most reputable dog training programs require evidence that the service animals they endorse have been put through an appropriate training program. Having video evidence that such a test has occurred is an excellent way to make sure that all the animals perform at an adequate level of discipline and behavior.

Chapter 2: The Three Factors that Define a Service Dog

This chapter introduces the legal definition of a service animal in the USA. Other countries have different laws and standards, and even within the USA the enforcement of the law varies widely.

A service animal *is not a pet*. The law requires that, for the purposes of access to the public, a service animal must be treated like a durable medical apparatus similar to a wheelchair or a pair of hearing aids. The Americans with Disabilities Act requires that people with disabilities be permitted equal access to all buildings where the public is allowed. Government buildings must therefore provide wheelchair ramps, automatic doors, and similar mechanisms that allow people to enter. New construction, be it for government, charitable, or private business purposes, must provide some means for differently abled people to enter, to conduct business as customers, or to function as employees. Even something as basic as a bathroom must be accessible to all different kinds of people. Furthermore, owners and operators of existing businesses or facilities must make a reasonable attempt to help people with disabilities gain access. They are not necessarily required to put in elevators or ramps—some older buildings simply cannot be retrofitted this way—but the law requires them to at least try to help people who want to do business.

Nobody can simply ban eyeglasses, leg braces, or hearing aids and still purport to do business with the public. To serve the public, a business has to serve the *whole* public—not just the portions of it that align with what the business owner or manager happens to favor. A service animal, for the purpose of the law, is in the same category as a walker or an oxygen tank. They simply can't be excluded from any place the general public is allowed, except for very limited situations I'll get to in a moment.

Contrary to popular belief, service animals do not have access rights to public spaces. *No* animal has the right of access. *People* have the right of access to public spaces, and in order to make use of those spaces they sometimes need medical equipment such as a service animal. The key word here is "need". To need a particular dog to accompany you as a service dog implies that you *have* a disability and that the animal has been *specially trained* to perform *tasks that are related to your disability.* ***These three things must be documented, or else in the eyes of the law they didn't happen.***

There are three factors required for an animal to be a service animal. The handler must have a ***documented disability***, the animal must be ***trained to perform specific tasks related to that disability***, and there has to be some *formal documentation, issued by a qualified organization,* that your animal has been trained to perform those tasks *and* meets minimum behavioral requirements for public access.

Factor #1: Documented Disability

A disability is a physical, emotional, or psychiatric problem that interferes with normal life activities. A *documented* disability is one that is recognized and acknowledged by a person who is medically qualified to make the diagnosis. To qualify your dog as a service dog, you must ensure your disability has been appropriately documented.

For hearing loss, necessary documentation of your disability could be in the form of a letter from your audiologist or ear/nose/throat specialist. It could be a copy of a recent hearing test which shows that your disability is significant. It could be a note from a child's pediatrician confirming a congenital middle ear deformity that results in hearing loss. Or it could be a note from an emergency room doctor confirming that you were in an accident that caused damage to your ears.

If you don't have documentation of your hearing loss, then as far as the law is concerned it doesn't exist and you don't have a disability. This standard of proof works wonderfully for people with mobility impairments or other disabilities that are obvious to observers. But it causes problems in the specific case of hearing loss, because we have to run the gamut, paying various audiologists, ENTs, physicians, and other doctors to look in our ears, say "I don't see anything", and send us a bill

12

along with a referral so that another medical professional can do the same thing.

Hearing loss often comes on gradually. Many people see it as part of getting old, and unless you have your hearing tested regularly because of a job requirement you may not notice the gradual deterioration. Hearing loss tends to go untreated in the United States, simply because insurance companies cannot afford to provide hearing aids for all the customers who need them. Hearing aids are expensive, they are not critical from a life-or-death perspective in the way that a Pacemaker is, and age related hearing loss is common enough to be considered normal. Therefore, most health insurance plans won't cover expenses related to hearing loss due to age. Some policies will provide hearing aids that are necessary due to accident or illness, but most insurance companies do everything they can to avoid holding up their end of the contract with the customer.

A person who doesn't have a documented disability is not eligible for a service dog. They might own a highly trained animal, but they do not need the animal to compensate for things their body or brain will not allow them to do. A diagnosis of congenital deafness, otosclerosis, or age related hearing loss can indeed qualify you to own a Hearing Ear dog. But if you don't have a written diagnosis by someone medically qualified to wield the appropriate rubber stamp, your dog will be a "pet" in the eyes of the law. Accordingly, one of the first things you need to do if you want a service dog is to *make sure your disability is documented*.

Many of the people who buy fake service vests online and put them on their pets to get away with bringing them onto an airplane or into a grocery store don't have a disability at all. Being a jerk doesn't count as a disability. Unfortunately, because many disabilities are invisible some individuals do get away with passing Rover off as a service dog. This creates problems for everybody.

Factor #2: Disability-Specific Training

The second factor that separates a service dog from a "pet in a vest" is disability-specific training. Your dog has to be trained to perform specific tasks related to your disability. If the animal in question has not been trained to perform specific tasks related to your disability, it's not a service animal.

There are some cute things that I've trained my dog to do, and some behaviors that have kind of developed through the normal course of my relationship with my dog. For example, Honeybits pulls my socks off for me in the evening, wakes me up when I'm having a nightmare, and comforts me if I've had a rough day at work. None of those tasks are related to my hearing loss so *they don't count*. Her door alerts, her siren alerts, her highly specialized nose licking behavior in response to a fire alarm, and the various alerts on alarm clocks, a ringing phone, and an unidentified intruder all count.

Notice that the behaviors that make Honeybits into a service dog are *trained* behaviors. They have been observed by a highly educated animal trainer, they have been captured on video, and they are the result of hours of deliberate work. An emotional support animal, whose sole function is to snuggle up and relieve the handler's unpleasant emotional state, does not have special trained behaviors related to a documented disability. As beneficial as they are, they don't count as service animals. Neither does an animal that is simply responding to his or her environment in a way that coincidentally provides useful information to the handler. A junkyard dog that barks and jumps when an intruder comes by may perform a useful alert function, but he or she is not a service animal.

Factor #3: Official Recognition

The third and final factor is official recognition. Unless you can get a reputable trainer to sign off on the specifically trained tasks, to administer the Public Access Test, and to certify that your dog has passed it (or to provide some other evidence that you and your dog should be out in public together), *your animal's skills and excellent behavior don't count.*

Proper training organizations provide proof of their endorsement. These proofs include vests, patches, and paperwork such as ID cards or official letters indicating that they have supervised the training and testing, and that they endorse your animal as a service animal. Every state has specific organizations (mostly charities) that they recognize as having trainers who are qualified to instruct service animals and their handlers.

There are several organizations that purport to certify or supervise individual trainers, charities, and private companies that perform service dog training. One of them is ADI, or Assistance Dogs International. ADI promulgates and distributes a version of the Public Access Test to their member organizations. However, as of this writing they focus on not-for-profit charities and not on for-profit trainers. A for-profit trainer or dog training company can be just as competent as a charity but they will not be recognized for ADI. Also, ADI focuses solely on the training process and on credentials. They do not audit their member organizations or vouch for their financial, ethical, or legal reliability. So, ADI membership isn't a guarantee that the training organization you're considering is honest or well run. Lack of ADI membership therefore isn't evidence that the trainer is incompetent. The best solution is to look for endorsement from the state or provincial authority.

Charitable, tax exempt, or not-for-profit status is not relevant to whether an organization is capable of adequately training a dog or of administering the Public Access Test. Whether a service dog comes from a private business or from a public charity is irrelevant to the quality of the training. The critical factor is that the certifying organization must have a standard Public Access Test, and they must maintain other standards related to vaccination, dog behavior, and documentation. They must be able to show that each animal they endorse has received an appropriate amount of training over a reasonable period of time, and that each animal meets minimum behavioral standards for public access.

Many tax exempt charities delegate the actual training and testing of the service dogs they find. The individual trainers might be freelancers, or they might be employed by a separate dog training company that has the charity as a customer, training the dogs and handlers that are found and vetted by the charity. The charity then handles the recruitment of the people with disabilities and of the dogs who will be trained to serve them, but the professional trainers are the ones who handle the hands-on aspect.

Why Pursue Official Recognition?

Getting official recognition for your dog requires effort and expense. You have to keep your vaccinations and licensure up to date, training is not free unless you qualify for a grant of some kind, and depending on where you live it can be difficult or expensive to find a qualified trainer.

There are lots of people who train their own animals to perform service functions, and if you're a Deaf dog owner I would bet my next paycheck that you've trained your dog—accidentally or on purpose—to do at least a few things that help get you through your day. Because Hearing Ear dogs do most of their work in the home, many Deaf people don't pursue any kind of official recognition. I think that's a mistake for the following reasons.

First, you may have to travel unexpectedly due to a family emergency and require the specific services your dog provides. If you aren't being given official credit for the work your dog does, you aren't going to be able to bring him or her along except as a pet—and pets aren't welcome everywhere.

Second, the public activities required to prepare for the Public Access Test will get you out and around with your dog. That's healthy for both you and your animal. It also helps your dog get used to the various places he or she will go with you, and teaches your dog to adapt quickly to new environments and situations.

Third, if anything happens to you and you don't know who will care for your Hearing Ear dog when you're no longer able to do so, a service dog or former service dog will have families lining up to take him or her in. You will never have to give your best friend to a shelter or to a stranger. Even if your animal is retired and no longer works as a service dog, a well-trained animal is a fantastic pet.

Why Are Pets in Vests a Problem?

Earlier in this chapter, I mentioned that bogus service animals create problems. Anyone can go online and buy a service dog vest or harness (and, when you have a service dog, that's a great way to get a harness that fits or that suits the season). But because service dog paraphernalia is for sale to everybody, there's nothing to prevent the average John or Jane Doe from buying professionally-made, high-quality regalia, complete with an official-looking ID card for the dog. When their pet is dressed up this way, there's nothing to visually distinguish him or her from a real service dog.

The problem with pets in vests is that they are seldom trained to operate in a high-stress environment. Walking around in public where there are all kinds of strange people, noises, smells, and other animals is stressful for animals who are used to an indoor environment or a dog run. A pet who doubles as a guard dog is by definition not socialized to be friendly toward strangers, and he or she may even be aggressive. A pet who is kept in a backyard run may not understand that urinating or defecating in a restaurant is bad form. Even a well-intentioned, friendly pet may jump up on a child or an elderly person, causing injury. There are places where pets are welcome, such as dog parks and pet-friendly stores. But outside these environments, the average pet is far too likely to bite, to damage property, or to behave disruptively.

When people pay to attend a concert or a movie, they expect to be able to listen to it without having their experience interrupted by a barking dog. When people pay for food, they expect to be able to eat it without having it snatched off their plate or out of their hands. When they pay to fly in an airplane, they expect to be able to do so without having to sit in animal urine or feces. People who must avoid animals due to allergies, fear, or simple dislike deserve to not be forced to interact with them. When the animal in question is a highly trained service dog, *nobody but the handler* is required to interact. The dog is trained to be quiet in public, to refrain from soliciting food or attention, and to avoid touching other people. A pet in a vest generally wants to interact and to seek attention from people or from other dogs. That's disruptive at best, and sometimes potentially dangerous.

There's a secondary consequence to people who have invisible disabilities such as hearing loss. Because so many idiots pass their pets off as service dogs, we are often publicly accused of doing the same. Nobody likes to be ridiculed, criticized, mocked, or rebuked by a stranger, especially in public. Anyone who has ever needed a placard or pass for a handicapped parking stall has probably experienced the ridicule of individuals who feel entitled to insult, belittle, or grill them about their medical conditions. It's not much different when you're out in public with a service dog, especially if your disability is invisible.

Sadly, there's a "more disabled than thou" element to society that believes that since *they* don't need help from a four-footed friend, you are somehow faking your disability or your need for an animal helper. If your dog isn't helping you at the moment, or if you don't need your dog to get groceries or to pump gas, it may be difficult for you to avoid people who are determined to harass you for having a "fake" service dog.

The world is also full of social justice warriors who get their kicks out of publicly challenging and grilling people who, in their opinion, aren't disabled or who are trying to pass off fake service dogs as real ones. They take pride in confronting you as you go about your business, attacting other people's attention to you, and sometimes even videotaping the encounter to be posted to a "callout" site on social media so that you can be humiliated in front of the whole world.

If you're nervous, or if you're a new team, you will be a magnet to the social justice warriors. They will do their absolute best to get you thrown out of a store or a public building when you and your service dog are just quietly going about your business. The slightest indecision, nervousness, or mistake on your dog's part will bring on the critics, and no amount of proof or evidence will satisfy them. In their minds, you are a fraud and a felon who deserves to be publicly humiliated and driven out of "their" space. They won't be satisfied until you leave, and would actually prefer that you never set foot outside your home. But their righteousness and their sense of self-entitlement is rooted in the fact that some people *do* fake their service dog credentials.

I've learned to give as good as I get with social justice warriors who make a habit of accosting strangers in public. Every time someone suggests or insinuates that Honeybits is a fake service dog, I respond by suggesting and insinuating that my accuser is a rapist or a child pornographer. If they object to being characterized as a felon, I use the same logic against them that they are trying to use against me, because if it's OK for them to publicly accuse me of a crime I haven't committed, they must have a deep and pressing need to be measured by the same standards and treated the same way. This is a level of hostility I don't enjoy experiencing when I do something as simple as go to a grocery store or museum. Pets in vests are one of the root causes. If there weren't so many of them, the social justice warriors would find somebody else to hassle.

Chapter 3: Limits to Service Dog Access

There are going to be places where you can't bring your Hearing Ear dog. There are also circumstances under which you and your service dog may be legally ejected or barred from businesses, public buildings, or other places. This chapter will discuss the limitations to your access rights with your Hearing Ear dog. It will also discuss the process by which other people may legally challenge you when you enter an area where non-service animals are not allowed.

Your Right to Swing Your Fist Ends Where Someone Else's Nose Begins

In real life, one person's rights are always balanced by the rights of others. People's rights are limited by the law at the point where the exercise of those rights harms, or can reasonably be expected to harm, somebody else. For this reason, the right to freedom of speech does not include the right to yell "Fire!" in a crowded movie theater where no fire is actually present. The right to consume alcohol does not include the right to operate a motor vehicle while drunk. In the specific case of a service dog, your right to have your dog with you is limited to situations in which the presence of your animal doesn't create a danger or risk to someone else.

Public safety trumps our access rights along with our right to bring a service dog along. Dog allergies are real, and so is the need for sterile operating rooms and clean food preparation areas. Whenever a dog's hair, dander, or presence poses a danger to others, it's legal to deny access. Honeybits doesn't belong in the clean room areas of a computer chip fabrication plant, in a restaurant kitchen, in an operating room, or on the flight deck of an airplane. However I also can't help but notice that all the places I just described are off limits to the general public too. If you are in surgery, even the closest members of your family must wait in the lounge or the recovery room. That includes your service dog.

In the state of Hawaii, which is rabies free, dogs and other animals are required to be placed in quarantine. There are exceptions for service animals, *if* you go through the right process. You cannot just hop off the plane and head for the nearest tiki bar. There's only one airport that can accommodate you—HNL in Honolulu—and you must be prepared. Your dog must have the right vaccinations and it's up to you to ensure the evidence is provided to the right officials far enough in advance of your travel date. If you fail to do this, you will be allowed to come and go freely in Hawaii, but your dog will be quarantined. This process is necessary to ensure that parasites, germs, and other diseases are not introduced into a very vulnerable ecosystem. It is an example of public safety requiring limitations to public access rights.

Private Property Really Is Private

In a private home, or in fact any privately owned location that is not accessible to the general public, the public access laws related to service dogs don't apply. This may sound like an arbitrary law, and there are some circumstances under which it could feel unfair, but it's an example of a homeowner's right to limit entry to people he or she wishes.

I also want to clear up a very common misunderstanding about just why a "private business" should be subject to regulation. It's quite popular these days to assert that a privately owned business should be free from regulations intended for the rules that govern others. Yet it turns out that the regulations have nothing to do with who owns the business or what their personal opinions or beliefs are, and everything to do with whether the business serves the public.

Private Homes

Although you have the right to walk into a grocery store with your dog, you don't have the right to do the same thing at your in-laws' house without their explicit invitation. Anyone who owns or rents a living space has the right to decide who else can come in, and under what circumstances.

I strongly recommend that you ask before bring your service dog to someone's home even when you're an invited guest. Your service dog is presumably well behaved, but there's always a chance that someone else's home contains an environment or component your dog simply hasn't been trained to handle. One obvious example is pets. Your dog might be OK with other dogs, but has he or she been socialized to get along with cats? Ferrets? A Vietnamese pot-bellied pig? Mice? Rabbits? A ball python? How about a hamster or a large parrot? Even if your dog is the mellowest creature in the world, your host's pets are very unlikely to have received the same level of training and socialization. They may freak out and behave in a completely unpredictable way.

Years ago, a friend of mine brought over her mid-sized service dog—some kind of Sheltie cross. The dog was very well trained and an excellent support animal for my friend, but my cat bolted in fear. The dog's chase instinct kicked in, and he yanked the leash out of my friend's hand to chase my cat around my home. My poor cat hid under the bed, but the dog still tried to follow him. It wasn't easy to contain the dog, and my cat was so traumatized by being chased around his home that he shook for hours. So, for that particular dog, my home wasn't a good environment. This surprised me, because other friends of mine had brought dogs to visit in the past and there had never been an incident. Their dogs, obviously, had less of a chase instinct and less aggressive behaviors toward cats. For whatever reason, this particular service animal had undergone significant training, including having passed his Public Access Test, without having had his chase instinct triggered. We found out that day that he was a great dog but that he had some limits when it came to being around other animals.

Private Clubs

A private club is a kind of business that is set up for some specific purpose such as recreation or socializing. It is jointly owned by its members, who share the operating expenses and who generally pay an introductory fee and regular membership dues. Examples of private clubs include golf and country clubs, private dance clubs, business networking clubs, and leisure clubs based on the English gentlemen's clubs of the 19th century.

The idea behind a private club is that its members have something in common such as a sport, a location, or a shared life experience of some kind. They band together to pay for a facility for their collective use so that they can meet and socialize with each other. In this respect, they are business partners because they jointly own the assets of the club. But their business does not serve the public: it exists only to provide services to its members.

Private clubs don't have to follow anti-discrimination or disability laws. They are not required to have wheelchair ramps, accessible bathrooms, or any other accommodation intended to help people with disabilities. They definitely don't have to allow wheelchairs or any other form of durable medical equipment on their property, and that includes service dogs.

The special exemption for private clubs comes from the fact that nobody can be forced to accept any other person as a business partner or co-owner of property. Housing co-ops are therefore within their legal rights to deny membership to people in categories they don't like. They therefore routinely reject single females and members of visible minorities. It's legal.

When it comes to a private club, a club's finances must be set up so that new members pay their fair share of the cost related to running the club plus a fair portion to compensate the existing members of the club for the start-up expenses. Private clubs therefore have processes by which they choose whether to accept or reject a prospective new member. Some casual dance clubs simply require that new "members" be sponsored by an existing member and that the new member pay annual dues for continued access. On the other end of the spectrum, an extremely exclusive tennis club may require an extensive background check, a credit check, and hefty annual fees.

Another way private clubs maintain their exclusivity is by requiring a majority vote among the existing members to accept or deny each new member. This means that even if there aren't any rules on the books about whether to admit a person of a different gender, race, religion, or political affiliation, members of an exclusive private club can and do keep "others" out simply by voting only for new members who resemble themselves. If no "outsider" is sponsored as a new member, or accepted by a majority vote, they all remain on the outside.

Given that non-discrimination laws don't apply to private clubs, it's easy to see how they could easily exclude a prospective member who has a service dog, or require that the dog not be brought to the club. Such clubs also have the right to refuse admission or accommodations to *existing* members who develop a disability. How often this happens is hard to determine because private clubs aren't usually forthcoming about what goes on behind closed doors, but there are clubs composed entirely of married people who deliberately kick out widows and widowers, so it's not too much of a stretch to imagine a newly injured or sick person being kicked out of a particularly snooty country club or refused access due to their service dog. If this happens to you, I'm very sorry that you're having a negative experience now, but it's part of the deal you made when you decided to pay money to hang out with jerks.

Shared Housing

If you're renting an apartment, you have the right to bring your service animal without being charged a "pet fee" or a higher rate of rent. Yet you're on the hook to replace anything your dog destroys or damages, including carpet "accidents". You must also make sure that you abide by the standards of conduct, which include obeying local noise ordinances and whatever house rules apply.

Very few people object to an occasional low woof or a playful yip, provided it's only once in a while and provided it doesn't happen when theya re trying to sleep. If your dog gets a toe caught in something and screams or freaks out, it's understandable because it's an involuntary reaction to something rare. But when the noise is voluntary and when it doesn't stop, it's going to irritate people. If your dog decides to join in a neighborhood howl-a-thon one evening and you end up with a noise complaint, it's up to you to ensure that it doesn't happen again. Your neighbors deserve peace and quiet.

Noise is a special issue for people in the Deaf or hard-of-hearing community. Those of us who still have some hearing tend to play our music and our televisions louder than a normal person does, simply so that we can hear them. We sometimes talk louder, we don't notice it when we let a door slam or bang pots and pans together in the kitchen, and people who live with us or socialize with us might sometimes have to speak loudly or even shout to be heard. We aren't always aware of it when the noise we make is loud enough to disturb others. When we live around other people, if we want to get along well with them we have to make sure to pay attention to what we're doing and to comply with other people's requests to dial down the noise even if we don't believe it's a problem. Our service animals may contribute to the noise in our households even if we aren't aware of it.

If you're in the market for an apartment or house, nobody can refuse to rent or sell to you based on the fact you have a service dog. They are entitled to request the appropriate documentation such as proof that you have a disability and that your animal has been approriately trained. Whether your dog is present has no effect on your neighbors because presumably the dander and pet hair is confined to your housing unit. This dynamic changes if other people are sharing the house.

If you're renting a room from a live-in landlord, if you've answered an ad for a roommate or house-sharing situation, or if you're booking a temporary rented house, the anti-discrimination laws do not apply. When people will be sharing the entry and common areas of the house with you, such as the living room, your dog's presence affects those people. If you relax on the couch for an hour with the dog at your feet, even if you vacuum up the pet hair afterwards the next person who sits on the couch is not in a dog-free environment. If they are allergic to dogs, *any* dog may trigger a reaction. Likewise, if your housemates already have pets that are not compatible with your dog, he or she is a no-go and the room in question is a bad fit for you.

Your right to have your service dog live with you does not trump other people's right to be safe and comfortable in their own home, or to live with people whose lifestyles are compatible with their own. Nobody can be required to share living space with an animal that makes them uncomfortable or that causes them medical distress.

"Private" Businesses, However...

Many people can't quite understand why a "private business" or a "privately owned business" should have to follow any laws in particular, including the laws related to service animals, handicap accessibility, non-discrimination, and the need to serve the entire public. The fact that the word "private" appears in the description of the business gives some people the idea that the people who own that business should have the same level of control over the business that they do in their homes. But that's simply not true.

The word "private", used in the context of "private business" refers to the means of ownership. A privately held business or corporation is owned and controlled by specific individual shareholders who do not have the right to sell or to redistribute those shares. A publicly held corporation, by contrast, has some or even all of its shares traded on a stock exchange. So, the local mom-and-pop grocery store may be a private business, whereas the supermarket across the street is a publicly held corporation. Yet they both serve the general public, and they frequently employ or do business with members of the general public as well. For this reason, various laws and standards come into play such as minimum wage laws and health codes.

The number of people who own or have shares in a business is irrelevant to whether that business has to follow the zoning, health, tax, or other laws that apply to other similar business. If you have a flower shop and own it as a sole proprietorship or limited liability company, you still have to follow the same fire code as the flower shop next door that is part of a national chain where shares in the parent company are traded on a major stock exchange.

Private businesses are required to follow the same rules for disability-friendly construction and business operations as any other kind of business. They aren't required to let you in anywhere a member of the general public isn't allowed to go, but unless the presence of your dog poses a risk to somebody there, they do have to let you in with your service animal.

Deaf Rights in Other Nations

Most North American and Western European countries have embraced service animals and have favorable laws, however it's important to do your research before you go. Most nations have laws requiring vaccination, and you will have to produce the proper records, sometimes in advance, for your dog to be allowed entry instead of being kept in quarantine. Your dog will not be exempt from vaccination or quarantine laws simply because he or she is a service animal. When your dog is in quarantine you will have to function without him or her.

Having a Hearing Ear dog does not override local law when it comes to restrictions on your driving privileges. Many countries, as you are no doubt aware, restrict the right of Deaf people to drive. In Japan, Deaf people have finally won the right to drive but are legally required to put a yellow butterfly sticker on their vehicle. Hey, at least it's not a six-pointed star... but it still says "look at me: I'm vulnerable, rob me first."

Having a Hearing Ear dog will unfortunately not help you avoid being treated as a second-class citizen when you travel. Not all nations have laws that require hotels or restaurants to accommodate your animal. So, you may end up eating outside or on the go a lot. Your dog may not be permitted on public transit or in taxis or private conveyances.

This doesn't mean you can't travel to places that are unfriendly to service dogs. You must simply accept that there will be more planning and expense required, and that you must have a plan to remain within the law and to avoid attracting negative attention during each part of your journey. It's a little bit like, say, trying to visit Saudi Arabia while female. There will be more regulations, more hoops to jump through, and more artificial legal barriers to your participation if you wish to do something as simple as book a hotel room or walk down a public street.

Chapter 4: Your Responsibilities

With rights come responsibilities. In general, your service dog is treated as an extension of yourself, except for some restrictions like the ones I described in the previous chapter. This chapter will describe some of the duties and legal responsibilities that go along with having a service dog. I think of them in two general categories: your duties to your dog, and your duties to other people.

Category 1: Your Duties to Your Dog

Your dog would literally die for you, in a heartbeat, without thinking the matter through or considering it a misfortune. Think about that for a second. You are loved unconditionally.

In exchange for your dog's tireless devotion, you've got some moral obligations to that animal. This section describes a few of them. In a nutshell, it's up to you to take care of your service dog's needs, and because we are redirecting so much of our animals' time and attention to serving us, we often take away time and energy the dogs would otherwise be using to care for themselves. If we don't make up the difference by ensuring our service dogs get what they need, *it won't happen.*

When you're out and around, you know how to look for a restroom when you need one, and you pick up something to eat or drink when you're thirsty or hungry. Your dog isn't at liberty to do that. When you're eating in a restaurant, your dog is at your feet *not* eating. When you stop at a drinking fountain or buy a bottle of water on a hot day, you dog doesn't have access to it. When you sit down at a bus station or in an airport, your dog is still on duty. After a few hours of this, the dog is going to be hungry, thirsty, tired, and probably in need of a potty break. If you aren't mindful of this, you will soon get a surprise you don't like.

Dogs can't speak, and they're respectful creatures overall, so you're not likely to hear: "Boss, you had a good restaurant meal and three glasses of water, we've walked for five miles in the heat, and you just went to the bathroom. When's it my turn?" Instead you'll get a puddle on the floor when you don't expect one, or a tired and thirsty dog who just needs a rest or a drink of water and who loses it when you walk by a fountain.

A good cowboy takes care of his horse before he takes care of himself. He doesn't take a drink of water unless his horse has been offered one first, and he doesn't eat until after he's fed his animal. That's a good policy for us too. First thing in the morning, I feed and water Honeybits and offer her the potty. When I come home from work, the very first thing I do is to walk the dog.

Another good general rule is that your dog is usually feeling what you're feeling. When you're hungry, your dog's hungry. When you're thirsty, your dog's thirsty. When you're tired, your dog is probably exhausted. When you need the restroom, so does your dog. If you have a small, short-haired dog, then if you're cold enough to need a sweater or jacket, your dog *really* needs to warm up.

Food and Water

Your dog is an animal, not a machine. He or she needs good quality food and consistent access to fresh water. In your home, you must provide your dog access to fresh water 24 hours a day, 7 days a week. When you're out and around, it's practical to bring a bottle of water. Many pet stores sell collapsible bowls or folding extensions that can allow any water bottle to become dog-friendly.

Food-wise, you may have to experiment a little to find the kind of food that is right for your dog. Depending on breed, size, and age your animal may need different types and amounts of food. Dry food is generally better for a dog's teeth because the chewing action helps keep the teeth clean. But for a growing puppy (if you're raising your own) it's physically impossible to overfeed a pup if you're supplying high-quality protein.

Small dogs eat less than large ones, but they tend to need to eat more frequently. The toy breeds can suffer from low blood sugar if they are not fed regularly. Your dog will benefit from either a regular feeding schedule or free access to food. If you're out and around, it's reasonable to keep a small plastic bag of food for your dog, and to offer it every hour or so or at regular feeding times, especially if you're doing something unusual such as traveling long distances.

It's a bad idea to feed "people food" to your dog. He or she is not a garbage disposal. Commercial food that is processed and fed to humans is unsuitable for animal consumption because of the high fat, salt, white starch, and sugar content. Although your dog does need some salt, the level of salt humans consider tasty is extremely unhealthy for dogs. The chemicals we use as preservatives do not appear to be harmful to humans in small amounts, but keep in mind that a dog is smaller than a human and that the long-term effects of large amounts of preservatives on dogs are not fully understood.

There are human foods that are extremely toxic to dogs. Grapes, raisins, and wine can be deadly and so can onions or garlic. Fruits such as cherries, apples, or apricots are fine as long as you remove the pits or seeds. Anything with active yeast in it should not be fed to a dog, and many people avoid sharing bread or cookies for this reason. Salty foods should be avoided because the dog instinctively drinks water to compensate for salt or zesty seasoning. Salt imbalance and the resulting water intake can throw off a dog's kidney function. If you have a small dog—and most Hearing Ear dogs are of small to medium size—the critical dose is much lower than it would be if the dog were bigger.

There's a trend in which people make special effort to feed their dogs raw meat instead of cooked meat. If you keep a regular schedule and can observe safe meat handling practices, and if your dog eats everything you put in front of him or her, feel free to go for an all-raw diet. I've never been able to do this safely, because Honeybits is a nibbler. She takes a few mouthfuls of food at a time, as she feels the need, throughout the day when we're home. I simply can't leave raw meat sitting in a dish all day long. But Honeybits appreciates a slice of red bell pepper, or a bit of boiled carrot or potato provided it is unsalted.

You don't need to buy the most expensive products on the market. There's nothing wrong with feeding your dog "byproducts" such as ground-up organ meats, ears, and lips, provided you make sure that the protein level isn't too low and the fat level isn't too high. Watch out for additives: many dogs don't do well with wheat, especially the genetically engineered kind that is popular in the United States right now. You don't have to go completely grain-free unless your dog is displaying signs of food intolerance such as watery eyes, scratching, or red patches on the skin.

There are people who prepare meals for their dogs out of eggs, chicken, and similar foods. These are best cooked, because you dog is just as susceptible to salmonella as you are. But with a much smaller body size than a human, a dog becomes dehydrated much more quickly than a human being and can die of food poisoning.

Your dog should not eat bones that are likely to snap and splinter. Chicken bones are notoriously bad for dogs. Rawhide chew toys are also relatively high-risk, but a good quality beef T-bone or soup bone shank is reasonable provided you supervise the dog and take the bone away if it starts to splinter.

Rest and Off-Duty Time

Animals, just like humans, need to sleep. Your dog needs to sleep more hours per day than you do. As crepuscular animals, dogs are instinctively more active in the morning and around sunset. These are the times he or she will want walks, play, and interaction with you. Late at night and during midday, your dog will tend to nap. This will not necessarily interfere with his or her Hearing Ear work in the home. Dogs don't sleep as deeply as humans, and if your dog is attuned to a knock at the door or a ringing phone, he or she will wake up and get to work.

To accommodate your dog's need for rest, make sure he or she has a soft, clean bed of some kind. Locate the bed in a quiet part of the house, but you may notice that your dog prefers to be in the same room as you if anything is going on.

Your dog shouldn't be "on duty" all the time. He or she deserves a little bit of time to play and to just be a dog. I give Honeybits a daily walk around the neighborhood, especially before I ask her to come out with me in public. This allows her to wake up, warm up, empty her bladder and bowels, and get ready for an adventure with me.

Potty

Bowel and bladder control is vital to service dog training. Some animals can learn to urinate or defecate on command, but not all of them can. (Can you? I never could.) But most animals have a daily routine or cycle of some sort. They have to "use the bathroom" after waking up, before or after eating, and after exercise. Dogs can avoid impacted anal glands and constipation if their handlers walk them to allow them to defecate after some exercise.

A dog who has a regular daily routine with a wake-up time that doesn't vary much will need to go outside in the morning at about the same time. Anyone who has raised a puppy is familiar with the early morning wake-up. If you let your dogs go outside into a yard or enclosed area to do their business, you may still benefit from other forms of potty training.

Because Honeybits weighs only about five pounds and our home is on the migration path for red-tailed hawks, I do not allow her to go outside unsupervised. I walk her and clean up with a poop bag. I've also trained her to use the little square "potty pads" many people use for their pups. The dog prefers gravel or dirt as a poop site, followed by grass, however I notice that when I'm traveling or in an urban environment there aren't always desirable poop spots. I have to make an extra effort to provide her with a safe potty location, and sometimes unfolding a potty pad on the floor of a gas station restroom is enough of a cue to remind her that she has an opportunity to empty her bowels or bladder.

Like human beings, dogs understand when they have to "go". Small dogs, or dogs who are drinking a lot of water due to the heat, have to urinate more often and eat or drink more often. We're accustomed to looking for restrooms for ourselves and to anticipating when we might have to go a long time without one, but our dogs simply can't plan ahead and anticipate the way we do. You have probably experienced the discomfort or outright pain of being stuck in a vehicle on a road trip with a full bladder but nowhere to stop. If so, you most likely learned to take advantage of every rest stop and to plan in advance so that there's a chance to use the restroom before you leave. Dogs don't usually draw conclusions like these. We therefore have to make time to take "potty breaks" for them. These should occur roughly every hour or so.

Unlike human beings, dogs seldom have an urge to urinate and defecate at the same time. A good ten-minute walk is sometimes enough to get a dog's system going, especially if you're driving somewhere and have stopped for some reason or another.

At some times during Honeybits's training process, I tried to take her out in public without "emptying the dog" first, or I allowed myself to get distracted enough to ignore the subtle signals my dog was giving me. I won't go into detail about the consequences of this decision except to say that it was messy, embarrassing, and completely preventable.

Empty the dog before you go out. Seriously.

Exercise

If it's hot or cold outside, check the temperature of the surface you're about to walk on. Understand that your dog is barefoot. If the pavement is too hot or too cold for you, it's too hot or too cold for your dog also. Make use of protective foot coverings for your animal. Understand that your dog can get sunburned or hypothermic. If you're going to spend time outdoors, put some sunscreen on the short-haired dog's ears or bundle the shivering pooch up in an appropriately sized shirt or jacket. If it's cold enough for you to want a jacket, your little Miniature Pinscher needs one too. If it's hot enough for you to be panting or sweating, your German Shepherd most likely needs a rest and a cold drink of water. Dogs can't sweat to cool off the way we can.

Medical Care and Grooming

Your dog needs to see a vet for regular vaccinations and check-ups. Dogs with medium and long hair need to be brushed. Depending on how long your dog's toenails grow and how much he or she walks around outside, you may need to trim your dog's nails. Most dogs need to be bathed regularly. You can do these things yourself, or you can pay a professional groomer to do them. But they have to be done.

Safety

You are responsible for your dog's physical safety. The fact he or she is considered durable medical equipment doesn't mean you can abuse or neglect your service dog without legal consequences. If you leave your service dog in a hot car, or refuse to provide necessary medical care, or allow children or family members to abuse the dog, you could face criminal charges for animal cruelty.

Most reputable trainers will recommend that you avoid dog parks because so many poorly trained and unvaccinated dogs hang out there. Your service dog is far too valuable to risk.

When you travel with your dog in a moving vehicle, you must secure him or her safely. For a Hearing Ear Dog who alerts me to traffic sounds, I have a special basket that allows her to interact with me and work while I drive. The basket fits over the passenger seat and contains a tether that attaches to her harness.

If you encounter an aggressive person or dog, you may have to physically protect your dog. Part of your training includes how to speak to other people who are behaving inappropriately toward your dog by trying to distract or pet him or her. You will also learn how to physically intercept an aggressive animal before it hurts your dog.

There are some places your dog simply doesn't belong. It's not that the dog is necessarily a danger to other people in the area, it's that the environment poses a risk to the dog. No dog belongs on a busy factory or slaughterhouse floor, on the deck of a crab boat, or up an electrical pole. If your work regularly requires you to be in such an environment and you truly can't function without a service animal at work, it's probably time to look for a different job.

The vast majority of a Hearing Ear dog's work is in the home, the car, the hotel room, or other private space. That's when you need the dog. If you work outside the home, there's a very good chance that you can make use of adaptations besides your dog. So your Hearing Ear dog isn't likely to help you much at work the way a Seeing Eye dog might help a blind person. You're still physically capable of getting around, and the things made difficult by your hearing loss (such as hearing spoken words) aren't things your dog can help you with. Most people with Hearing Ear dogs leave them at home while they work.

Travel presents a separate set of safety challenges. Having a Hearing Ear dog definitely helps me with siren and horn alerts while in a car, and her ability to wake me up in response to a fire alarm will save my life the next time such an alarm goes off in a hotel while I'm asleep. But when most people vacation, they make day trips to local attractions. So, if you're traveling to a noisy, chaotic environment such as a theme park, do you really need your dog to be present? Would he or she be happier and healthier napping in the hotel room and guarding your suitcase? Do you have some other means to get by in the theme park, such as the presence of friends and family members? Have you access to public or group transit to and from the hotel? If you don't need your dog *at* the theme park and you don't need the dog to *get* to the theme park, it's OK to let him or her relax at the hotel and have some time off.

Long-Term Care

If you are lucky, you and your dog will have many mutually rewarding years together. But human lifespans are longer than dog lifespans, and the time will most likely come when your service animal can't work anymore and must retire. It is your duty to provide care for him or her as long as he or she wants to live with you, and to provide medical care as needed. In the end, if your dog is suffering and no longer has a good quality of life, it's up to you to ensure your dog is euthanized humanely. Don't just leave him or her in the hands of a vet tech: stay with your loyal dog to the end.

If for some reason you are not physically capable of caring for an aging animal, make sure that you discuss this contingency before acquiring a service dog. The organization that trains your dog may be able to advise you.

Sometimes, due to accident or disease, we die before our animals do. Have some intelligent plan about what you want to have happen to your service animal if you predecease him or her. Make sure you know who the animal's caregiver is going to be, and do something to ensure that he or she has the money to feed your service dog and to provide for his or her needs once you're gone. This could take the form of an insurance policy payable to your dog's caregiver, or you may use a will or trust to provide for your animal.

Category 2: Your Duties to Others

This section deals with your duties to other human beings. Other people are generally more than willing to compromise and to not make trouble over your service dog, but it's important to be mindful and considerate of them in exchange.

Liability

You are legally and financially accountable for any damage your dog might do, no matter what the reason. If your dog chews up linoleum in the apartment you've rented, you're on the hook to pay to repair the damage. Failure to do so will result in a lawsuit and a judgement against you. The fact your animal is a service dog *is not a defense against civil or criminal liability for what the animal does.*

A well-trained service animal does not bite people or other animals. Many do not bite or snap even in self-defense. In fact, if your service dog were to bite another animal or a person, that dog would have to be retired unless you could show the authorities that you or the dog were actually being attacked by an animal big enough to do damage. You would also be required to pay for treatment for any injuries to other people or to their animals.

Challenge and Response

As a condition of being allowed to bring your service dog into areas generally accessible by the public, you must be prepared to answer polite questions about your animal within the limits of the law.

In the United States, there are only two questions business owners or employees are allowed to ask:

(1) Is that a service animal? and

(2) What services has the animal been trained to provide?

In the case of a Hearing Ear dog, your answers would be "yes" to the first, and for the second you would say: "my dog alerts me to things around me that I cannot hear." If you're in the mood, you can list a few.

You don't actually have to tell the questioner that you're Deaf or hard of hearing, and it's illegal for people to ask what your disability is. However, since hearing loss is an invisible disability it may be useful to point to a hearing aid or a cochlear implant pickup to support your statement.

You are not legally required to dress your service dog in a vest or harness, or to carry an ID card or a portfolio with the dog's credentials. Most people prefer to do this, simply because even legal challenge questions get old after a while. There may be times when you don't feel like talking to anyone, or when you're busy with an important text. If you simply want to read quietly, people may not be able to get your attention by speaking to you. There's a subset of the population that feels entitled to touch you, grab you, or shake you when they want your attention. Or they might just decide to mess with your dog or to lecture you. A service vest won't prevent accusations of having a "fake service dog", especially not from people with preconceived notions about what a service dog should look like in terms of size or breed.

I myself am not a fan of the portfolio approach. It was necessary during Honeybits's training, because she had not yet earned her service dog vest and was wearing the same kind of ordinary harness anyone can buy at a pet store. It included proof of my hearing loss (in case the hearing aids I was using at the time weren't convincing) and a letter from Duke City Dog Academy establishing that they were supervising Honeybits's training. Some businesses, museums, and public spaces allowed us in. Others did not. When I visited the Rosa Parks museum in Montgomery, Alabama in the summer of 2018, it had a huge sign on its door saying: "guide dogs only". An alert dog is technically not a guide dog. While the law does require equal access for all different types of service animals—the irony of a civil rights museum being publicly committed to inequality was not lost on me—I really wasn't in the mood for an argument so Honeybits and I just quietly slipped away.

I want to take this opportunity to praise the USS Alabama Battleship Memorial Park for their openness and welcome when the woman in charge of operations graciously allowed us full entrance and access rights. If you're ever in Mobile, Alabama with your service dog—even if he or she is only a trainee—I recommend that you visit the USS Alabama. They make special effort to be disability-friendly. Parts of the battleship are wheelchair friendly, and there's a gigantic indoor and outdoor selection of military aircraft and vehicles that you can see and touch. From time to time there's a book signing by a veteran or a military author. Honeybits and I also had the honor of meeting the retired Colonel Glenn D. Frazier, a legendary survivor of the Bataan Death March. We bought a signed copy of his book *Hell's Guest*, which I recommend to any student of history.

Documentation

You must keep your animal's records up to date. Vaccinations must be current and never allowed to lapse. If you live in a town or city that provides animal licenses, you must register your animal. Service dog licenses are generally free or low-cost.

If you are out with your dog in public, you must ensure he or she has the appropriate harness, vest, or other identifying garments with the necessary patches and ID card that identify your dog as a service animal. You must respond to the two legal questions ("is this a service animal?" and "what tasks is the animal trained to perform?") truthfully and politely. The harness and challenge responses are not technically a legal requirement, however I've noticed that if I want to be *welcome* wherever I go with Honeybits, I've found that it helps to behave like the kind of mature, considerate human being that other people want to have around. So, I meet people halfway by answering questions politely and by dressing Honeybits in proper attire.

Credible Behavior

It's your job to ensure that your service animal acts like one when you're out in public together. You must not allow the dog to play with people, run around off-leash, bark, or urinate or defecate inappropriately. As I mentioned earlier, I find it useful to have a short walk with Honeybits "off duty" before taking her out, so that she can comfortably do her business, sniff things, and just be a dog for a few minutes before dressing up and getting to work. Making potty in a parking lot is fine provided you clean it up. Making potty in a museum or store is not OK.

In general, service dogs aren't carried around unless you have to take them up or down a ladder or unless the type of work they provide requires that they be next to you. The rule is "four on the floor": four paws on the ground, and walking around. The animal is not carried in a body sling unless there's a valid medical reason to do so, and a Hollywood-style purse is simply out of the question. However, my dog's safety takes precedence and I'm not about to put a very important and expensive investment at risk just to provide someone else with the visual image they're looking for. If there's broken glass on the ground or anything else that creates an immediate hazard for my dog, I can and do pick her up and carry her through it. I've used the "emergency pop-up" to rescue Honeybits from large, aggressive unleashed dogs and from a large truck that began to suddenly back up while we were crossing behind it in the French Quarter of New Orleans. I've picked Honeybits up when she's stepped on a thorn or if the pavement is simply too hot for her to walk on, such as in some parts of the US south at midday in the summer. During her training, when she obviously did not have service dog credentials and was a trainee, some of the museums and public buildings believed they had the right to refuse us entrance due to her trainee status. State laws do vary from place to place. Yet a few of them compromised with me: we could see the museum, provided I carried the dog. This wasn't to prevent her from doing anything inappropriate. It was part of an explicitly negotiated compromise and a way of *proving* that she didn't do any damage.

Planning

If you are going to another country or traveling by air, it's your responsibility to learn and understand the rules of the place you're going. If you expect to be in a situation where your needs conflict with someone else's, it's your duty to help resolve the conflict instead of bone-headedly insisting on your rights. This isn't a legal requirement so much as a way to avoid hassle and inconvenience for yourself and others.

During the training process, you will gradually integrate your dog into public places, training him or her to behave appropriately. The goal is to gradually increase the distractions and complexity in your dog's environment until his or her obedience is strong enough to allow you to go into a grocery store, art gallery, or theater with the dog and not have the dog act out. It is completely reasonable for your training to include travel, however when you travel with a dog who DOES NOT yet have full service dog training and credentials (and this includes the phase while your dog is in training), that dog may not necessarily have the same rights as an animal who has passed the Public Access Test and who is already trained. I say "may not" because until your dog is officially a trainee, he or she is a pet and will most likely be treated as such by airlines and travel authorities.

Many regions, and most states, require that businesses and public places to allow access *for the purposes of training*. It's easy to tell the difference between someone who's training a dog and someone who's enjoying a vacation. When Honeybits and I were in a store or a restaurant with our trainer during the training process, Honeybits wore a vest and was very clearly being commanded, trained, and clicked at. A trainer was present, providing instruction. There was a clicker and a pocket full of dog treats. I didn't just wander in with a not-yet-fully-trained dog in a vest and say: "Hi, here's my service dog."

During Honeybits's training, my personal rule was that if I was out on my own on an errand or vacation, she traveled as a pet. Unless I had an explicit invitation to bring her somewhere (such as aboard the USS Alabama), issued by someone who had the authority to make the invitation, I brought Honeybits only to places where all well-behaved dogs are welcome. I took her to dog-friendly businesses such as pet stores or pet-friendly hardware stores. At restaurants, we dined only on the dog-friendly patios. I never entered grocery stores or restaurants with her unless my trainer was present and Honeybits was wearing what I affectionately called the "puppy bikini" with her service dog patch on it. We stayed exclusively in dog-friendly hotels or where she was already written into the timeshare contract.

Even in pet-friendly locations such as national parks, you can't bring a pet into a public building such as a restroom. The exemption given to service animals doesn't apply. So, you need another person to hold the dog's leash while you perform basic tasks like using the restroom or buying food or water. That's fine if you're traveling in a group (and are less likely to need the services your animal provides), but it's a gigantic problem when you're alone. You have only one pair of hands and can be in only one place at a time.

Traveling solo with a trainee service dog is a Catch-22. Even something as simple as emptying your bladder becomes logistically impossible unless you're willing to leave your dog alone in a hot car "for a few minutes" while you use the toilet. If you're delayed even slightly because of a long restroom line or some other unexpected event, your dog could be in medical distress or even dead by the time you get back. Or, if you do return in the expected three to five minutes, some do-gooder may have smashed in your car window to "rescue" your dog. If you need the services your dog provides, leaving the dog at home isn't an option.

Most campsites don't allow you to just tie your dog to a post or a tree while you set up your tent, because there have been too many people in the past who leave their dogs unattended but tied up for hours at a time. If you own a RV or tent, your dog can be in it while you run to the shower or restroom facilities, but obviously you need to set your accommodations up first. So, when I camped, Honeybits waited in the car until the tent was ready.

Being allowed to bring the dog into a restroom is a major blessing because you don't have to choose between your dog's safety and whether you get to empty your bladder. The snarky advice of "just leave the dog at home" is only viable for people who don't need the services the animal provides, who don't believe people with disabilities should shop or travel, or who don't understand that the only way to accustom a dog to a store or similar environment is to actually be in it.

Cleanup

Dogs pee and poop, just like we do. It's your job to clean up any mess your animal makes. Service dogs don't mindlessly lift a leg anywhere they please, but they do have bodily functions and you need to make sure they relieve themselves in an appropriate way. You must clean up the results. If you're out with your dog, you should have some wipes and a poop bag, just in case there's an accident or your errand takes longer than you expect and you need to give your dog a potty break outside.

It is never acceptable to leave your dog's poop on the ground instead of gathering it up. Doing this is considered irresponsible and poor form even for a pet owner, but it reflects only on the individual who fails to clean up after the pet. When a service dog handler fails to clean up, people who are already hostile to service animals or people with disabilities use it as a reason why we, or our dogs, shouldn't be allowed in public.

I have trained Honeybits to make use of a puppy pad for travel purposes. I open the pad up inside a restroom stall and she takes care of her business while I take care of mine. For a larger dog that may not be an option.

Chapter 5: What Hearing Ear Dogs Do

This chapter focuses on the specific services and behaviors provided by Hearing Ear dogs.

Hearing Ear dogs are a type of service dog trained to assist people who are Deaf or hard of hearing. They are categorized as "alert" dogs because the specific way in which they assist us is by *alerting* us to important things in our environment.

Trained animals, including service dogs, can be classified based on the kind of work they do. There are dogs that perform guiding behaviors (such as guide dogs for the blind), tracking and detection behaviors (such as search and rescue dogs), and herding behaviors. There are physical working dogs such as the Huskies that pull sleds and the fleet hunting dogs that lead hunters to their quarry. Many of today's breeds were developed for some purpose or another, and although some of the original tasks (such as bull-baiting) are now obsolete, the shape and attributes of the dogs trained to perform them make the dogs useful for other tasks. A brawny "pit bull" (a term which may refer to several different kinds of terriers or bulldogs and their crosses) is an ideal dog for a veteran with Post-Traumatic Stress Disorder (PTSD) or for a child who needs a strong, rock-like wall of muscle to brace against as he or she climbs into a wheelchair. But for Deaf or hearing-impaired people, a service animal helps by responding to sounds in the environment and informing the handler. This is called "alert" work. This chapter covers the kind of alert work that Hearing Ear dogs perform.

The "alert" category of working dog covers a broad spectrum of behavior. An alert behavior is one in which the animal notices something significant in his or her environment and uses a specific behavior to inform his or her handler. The earliest alert dogs were watchdogs who would raise an alarm if a suspicious person or animal came too close to the tent or the cave. The watchdog's function was not to attack, but to alert the humans in the area.

To a professional trainer, a Hearing Ear dog who wakes his or her handler up when a fire alarm is ringing is in the same category as a watchdog. So is a Seizure dog who notices small changes in the handler's heart rate and posture and warns the handler of an impending seizure. All alert behaviors are variations of the same process: the dog recognizes something in your environment you need to know about and takes a specific action to draw your attention to it. These behaviors may include pointing with the nose or body, nudging you to get your attention and then walking toward the source of the noise, or deliberately waking you up in response to an alarm clock, fire alarm, or ringing phone. These are highly reliable, trained behaviors that go significantly beyond a dog's natural reaction to an unexpected sound or event (although taking advantage of the dog's natural response is indeed the starting point for the training).

Directed Attention Seeking

According to Alexandra Horowitz in her bestselling book *Inside of a Dog*, dogs have been selectively bred by human beings for thousands of years. The dogs selected for breeding tend to be the ones with attributes or behavioral traits people find desirable. Among these traits is a strong desire for human attention. Dogs—notes Horowitz—look at us, watch us, and attempt to interact with us especially if they have imprinted on human beings as caregivers or members of their "pack". Attention seeking is normal for dogs. It's a very rare dog owner whose dog never brings a favorite toy for a game of fetch or tug-of-war, or whose reading or TV watching is never interrupted by a nudge, a bark, or the introduction of a furry nose in his or her line of sight. Alert behavior contains, by definition, attention seeking behavior. Yet it is not frivolous or random attention seeking: it is attention seeking with a *purpose*. I therefore sometimes refer to alert behavior as *directed* attention seeking.

Detection, Assessment, and Response

Every alert behavior consists of three phenomena: detection, assessment, and response. The first step in the process, detection, is the one that replaces our missing hearing.

Dogs hear (and see, and smell) all kinds of things that human beings can't. They pick up on things that range from the hum of an insect to a knock on the door or the sound of a child riding a bicycle along the sidewalk outside. Not all of these sounds, of course, represent a potential threat or even something the dog's handler needs to know about. An untrained dog might regard the garbage truck as the most interesting sound of all simply because a garbage truck smells like a lot of things that might be good to eat or to roll in. By contrast, a high-pitched beeping noise might seem insignificant or uninteresting. It takes training to teach a dog which sounds or phenomena are important to the handler—and likely to produce a reward if the dog responds appropriately.

Assessment is the process by which a dog determines whether the thing he or she hears is something the handler considers important enough to merit petting or even a treat. There can be two outcomes to this decision: the stimulus is important enough to merit an alert, or it is not. The dog must reliably guess correctly in *both* cases. It's not enough for a dog to perform an alert behavior in response to a stimulus the handler considers important: he or she must reliably refrain from "false alarm" behavior in which the dog performs the same behavior when the stimulus is not actually present. To be well trained, the dog must *not* alert on things the handler considers irrelevant, harmless, or unimportant. The pigeon perched on the windowsill or the squirrel in the tree outside, for example, are not things the handler needs to know about. A well trained watchdog, therefore, does not bark at a squirrel as though it were an intruder. Nor, for that matter, does a Hearing Ear dog.

The final step in the alert process is the response. The dog performs a specific act intended to convey information to the handler. It could be a movement, a sound, or a change in position. The dog signals to the human in a deliberate attempt to communicate. For a Hearing Ear dog, the alert is usually visual or tactile instead of a bark or other vocalization.

Far Beyond the Natural Behavior

All dogs communicate, or attempt to communicate, with one another and with us. They engage in attention seeking acts all the time. In fact, it may have been the canine tendency to seek attention and to communicate information with early humans that made wolves valuable as domestic animals. But the behavior displayed by an alert dog goes far beyond natural behavior.

Many families have "watchdog" animals that are not specifically trained to guard the home and yard, but that accomplish that goal simply by using their superior hearing and night vision to notice the things that we can't and to raise an alarm. This is definitely an alert behavior but service work requires more refinement. A watchdog that barks is perhaps a deterrent to a burglar, but what if the watchdog didn't bark? What if, instead, the watchdog came to the handler, woke the handler up, pointed the handler in the direction of a threat, and let the handler decide whether to make noise, sneak away, or attack? Stealthy detection and silent alerts are far more sophisticated than mindless barking. This more sophisticated behavior is what Honeybits displays.

Honeybits has four different "door" alerts, some of which are silent and some of which have a component intended to engage or describe the person on the other side of the door. The first alert is for my daughter alone: when she lets herself into my house, Honeybits quietly points and moves in her direction, nudging me awake at night if necessary. The second alert is for a stranger: one single bark at the door, followed by an attempt to come get me if necessary. The third alert has no bark but a series of wags, gurgles, wiggles, and chortles when a familiar friend is present. The fourth alert occurs only when someone is trying to break in.

Having seen Honeybits in action with Alert #4, I hope I never have to hear that again. The dog I've facetiously described as an "eighteen-inch subwoofer" produced some amazing bass notes that should not have been mechanically possible from a creature weighing only about five pounds. I've lost most of my hearing in that range, so the volume I heard must have been incredible. Honeybits roared and snarled like an angry Rottweiler until I opened the door to politely confront the stranger, who was in the act of trying my lock. No sooner did the door open than Honeybits stopped pretending to be a much larger dog and glared quietly. That gave me an opportunity to lie coolly to the intruder about "the big one". The intruder immediately left the neighborhood and never came back. (Good Chihuahua!)

Honeybits's intruder alert talents don't revolve around doors and windows. While tent camping in a deserted campground in Arkansas one night, she spontaneously came up with the "silent alert" I described earlier: every time an unfamiliar person or vehicle approached our tent, she woke up, pawed silently at my face until I woke up, and then pointed with her entire body in the direction of whatever was coming. This advance notice gave me one to two minutes during which I was free to whip out a camera with low-light enhancement, identify whatever was coming, and figure out whether I wanted to do a quick fade out the tent's rear door, confront, fight, capture, ambush, or even snipe. (*Very* good Chihuahua!) So although my tiny dog and I were alone in a stereotypical horror movie setting, we had a grand time. Had Jason Voorhees approached the tent, the movie would have ended in the opening scene.

If a "good" natural watchdog can be compared to a lightweight Toyota, Honeybits is a pointy-eared Maserati. There are reasons why she's this way, and most of them have to do with the hundreds of hours of work—and the thousands of dollars of professional training—that have been invested in her.

Distinctions from Other Types of Service Work

An Alert dog typically does not perform guiding tasks to physically move the handler from one place to another (as with a Seeing Eye Dog). Bracing, wheelchair pushing, or other tasks that require strength are not necessary. An Alert dog might carry seizure medication or hearing aid batteries, but they generally don't need to carry an oxygen tank or to pull a wheelchair. Physical deterrence of other people entering the handler's space, such as with a PTSD dog, is not in the scope of what a Hearing Ear dog is expected to do. Confrontational behaviors such as the ones displayed by the highly disciplined *Schutzhund* or "protection dogs", although they are highly valued by the police and military, are likewise out of scope. Most reputable trainers will not accept a dog for training if he or she has received protection training although agility or trick training is acceptable.

Disability Specific Services

This section is a breakdown of the particular services a Hearing Ear dog can be trained to provide. A few of them have become obsolete due to the invention of new technology such as cellular phones. Depending on your needs, not all of the trainable behaviors are necessary. Most people with Hearing Ear dogs select a subset of the available behaviors. Furthermore, exactly what your dog is trained to do in response to the stimulus will vary depending on what your needs are. The training of a Hearing Ear dog is therefore customized to suit you and your lifestyle. To be considered a service dog, your Hearing Ear dog should have at least four trained behaviors related to your disability.

The following lists include things you might want to train your Hearing Ear dog to do. The exact behaviors you select will depend on your lifestyle. Not everyone has a baby or a small child at home, and not everyone commutes by driving. Likewise, although most of us do cook or prepare food at home, not everyone has to function in a high-distraction environment such that food may boil over on the stove. Accordingly, a handler will work with a trainer to determine what kind of assistive behaviors the service dog must learn.

Typically a service dog performs at least four trained behaviors related to compensating for your disability. Depending on the extent of your hearing loss and how much independence you wish to have or to retain, you may select more behaviors, or fewer. You may even think of some that aren't on this list. Honeybits performs about nine of these specific assistive behaviors.

Indoors (at home, in a hotel, or any other place)

- Alert you to the presence of somebody at the door
- Use specific behaviors to inform you of who is at the door (family, stranger, etc.)
- Wake you up when a fire alarm sounds
- Wake you up when a clock radio or alarm clock sounds (partially obsolete: we now have alarm clocks that flash or vibrate, although these are not always available while traveling)
- Signal you when the baby is crying
- Alert you when something boils over on the stove
- Alert you to a fire elsewhere in the house
- Signal you when the microwave beeps
- Alert you to the presence of an intruder
- Point to a phone that is ringing (obsolete: we now have cell phones that vibrate or flash)
- Carry a note to a family member (obsolete: we now have cellular phones)

In the car

- Point in the direction of a siren or emergency vehicle
- Nudge you when a passenger is trying to speak to you (not always a desirable behavior and may be distracting)
- Get your attention when you become noticeably drowsy and should no longer drive (this can be built on the things a dog does out of the

desire to crawl over and nap with you, or it can be a behavior such as yawning that grows out of a mutual bond and that is reinforced during the training process)

On foot

- Make sure you are aware of someone approaching behind you
- Watch your back while you are distracted (such as when you use an ATM)
- Make sure you are aware of a dropped object such as your keys
- Carry your spare hearing aid batteries (not a trained behavior—just tuck them into a pocket of the dog's vest—but it's still very useful)
- Notify you when someone calls your name or tries to get your attention

While camping or traveling

- Alert you silently to a person or animal approaching your campsite
- Perform the same long-range identification of different categories of people that the dog would perform in your home
- Perform the same alarm clock or fire alarm alerts as would be appropriate in your home

In an airplane

- Wake you up when the flight attendant, or another passenger, is trying to get your attention
- Deter unwanted touching or physical contact from strangers

At school

- Alert your child when a distant person calls his or her name by stopping and pointing in the direction of the person trying to get your attention
- Notify your child of a dropped object, and possibly pick it up and carry it back
- Nudge your child when a teacher is trying to get his or her attention, so that teachers and school administrators don't feel the need to physically grab, shove, or touch your child to get his or her attention

How a Hearing Ear Dog Communicates

It's a common misconception that Hearing Ear dogs bark in response to something you need to know about. Barking makes no sense. Those of us who are profoundly Deaf can't hear a barking dog in the first place, and those of us with progressive hearing loss will gradually lose the ability. Furthermore, barking is a disruptive behavior that is unwelcome in public spaces such as movie theaters or restaurants. We therefore train our dogs to prefer subtler communication techniques when telling us what we need to know. We do this by selectively rewarding some of the dog's natural communication processes.

According to Alexandra Horowitz in her bestselling book *Inside Of a Dog: What Dogs See, Smell, and Know*, dogs have many ways of communicating with one another and with the human beings who occupy their world. These ways include changes of posture, touching, licking, and emitting odors. Dogs also have a wide range of vocalizations. When my hearing aids are turned all the way up and Honeybits is close by, I am astounded by the various chirps, squeaks, and clucks she makes while playing or while snuggling with me in the evening. One of the saddest things about my gradual hearing loss is that her subtle warbles and murmurs will eventually be beyond my ability to pick up no matter how much amplification I use. She can still sometimes get my attention with a single woof, if there's no background noise. But I find that she doesn't use it much. Perhaps it's because she's been with me since puppyhood. Back then, when she needed to empty her bladder at night, she'd gently tap my face with her paw. Nowadays, when she really needs to communicate with me she'll bump my leg or foot with her nose or paw. She has a vast array of nonverbal cues: the sideways wiggle she makes with her lower body when she needs to go to the bathroom, the way her ears perk up as her nose darts, arrow-like, toward the source of an oncoming siren, and the way she's been trained to respond to a shrill fire alarm by licking my nose.

An alert behavior is a deliberate behavior, and for a Hearing Ear dog the behaviors we select as special alerts fall into two categories: the visual, and the tactile. Auditory behaviors aren't useful for Hearing Ear dog purposes, and although dogs communicate with one another by scent, we cannot. Even if we had the olfactory sophistication to pick up on more than "remind me not to give the dog cheese again", scent signals provide information chiefly after the fact instead of the real-time alert behavior we need. Human beings have other kinds of after-the-fact communication. We tend to prefer sticky notes, text messages, or social media postings instead of piles of steaming dung (although, given the content of some social media, this may not be the best analogy.)

Visual Alerts

A visual alert is a change in position, posture, or configuration. Most visual alerts are exaggerations of normal dog communication signals. We're all familiar with wagging as a sign of satisfaction or contentment, and with a droopy head and tail as a sign of submissiveness or fear. But other movements ranging from a raised paw to an ears-up posture can be rewarded and exaggerated to provide a signal that is slow and obvious enough for us to catch.

When Honeybits suddenly turns her head to look at the source of an oncoming siren and deliberately orients her head and body toward it, she's pointing. Pointing is a posture change that sometimes involves a direction change. Some dogs point with the nose and with a raised paw. This is an exaggeration of an instinctive behavior that dogs use to direct one other's attention to distant objects. Dogs can learn to follow our gaze or our pointed fingers, but it takes a while because with our flat faces we're not nasally gifted enough to point our noses anywhere. It's relatively easy to tell what a dog is looking at: just follow the nose.

A standing or sitting posture can be a visual alert. Two of Honeybits's door alerts have a position component (along with an auditory component for whoever is on the other side of the door). The "stranger" alert requires her ears to be up, her tail to be up but not wagging, and for her shoulders and front legs to be rigid and erect. If she can stand on the windowsill next to the door to see better and to look taller, she will. She sometimes utters a single low-pitched "woof". That's not for me so much as for the other person. After this display, she will come find me if necessary and lead me to the door and assume her posture again. This behavior requires a change in both posture and position.

The most extreme change of position is when a dog runs through your visual field. Although our eyes are not as motion-sensitive as a dog's, running to enter your visual field is one way to get your attention from a distance prior to pointing or leading you.

When Honeybits has to empty her bladder or bowels, she wiggles and hunches her pelvis slightly forward. If I happen to be indoors, this is a signal to me to find a restroom and deploy a puppy pad or to take her outside. When she is dissatisfied with the water in her bowl, she leads me to the bathroom, jumps up at the tub faucet, and licks at it. The faucet does not drip, but I know from her series of movements that she is

49

communicating about water. Her food bowl is seldom empty, but if it is and she's hungry she will bat or tug at it.

Dogs have been known to suggest a walk by bringing a leash, or to initiate a game of fetch by bringing a ball. These are forms of visual communication. Other alert-related changes in posture may include abruptly sitting, lying down, or making a specific paw movement. These signals are frequently used by search-and-rescue or detection dogs.

Tactile Alerts

A tactile alert is one in which the dog communicates by touch. The dog may bump you with a shoulder or with his or her nose. Tapping your foot, ankle, knee, or face with a paw is a useful signal. The more intense or sustained the contact, the more urgent the message.

One of Honeybits's tactile alerts involves the smoke alarm. This is the one key alert that she absolutely has to get right, because it is a life-and-death emergency. Modern construction materials are so flammable that if you're in a burning building you have only a few seconds to get out. When the smoke alarm goes off, Honeybits is trained to come find me, jump up on me if I am asleep, and violently lick my nose. This is something you wouldn't ordinarily allow a dog to do. It's disgusting. Honeybits's tongue extends almost two inches beyond the end of her muzzle, and it's narrow enough to fit completely up my nostril. She can even open her mouth and come in at an angle to get more depth. So, no matter how deeply I'm sleeping, a doggy tongue up the nose captures my full and undivided attention. It's the most obnoxious thing she can do short of biting me, so it's the behavior I chose for the smoke alarm.

When the alarm clock goes off or if my phone rings while I'm asleep, Honeybits bats at my face with her paw. If there is someone at the door and she cannot get my attention by dashing by, she will press her nose into the side of my ankle. She also taps me with a toy to initiate a play session. If she wants my attention while I am seated at a table, she stands on her hind legs and taps me on the side of my knee with her paw or nose.

There are some natural dog behaviors that don't make good tactile alerts. Gently nipping or pretend-biting, for example, is misunderstood and can be interpreted as a threat. Similarly, jumping up on a person, scratching, and digging behaviors are bad choices for tactile alerts because they can injure a child or an elderly person.

Chapter 6: Selecting a Hearing Ear Dog

Not every dog is service animal material. Many animals that make outstanding pets are unable to function outside the home. You can adapt your home environment quite well to suit a pet with special needs, but it's impossible to adapt public space. Although most of a Hearing Ear Dog's work *will* be in the home, to qualify as a service animal in any state the dog must pass what's known as the Public Access Test. This test, which takes a couple hours to administer, consists of many different behaviors such as getting into and out of a car, behaving politely and unobtrusively when encountering other people, and controlling the impulse to greet people or to solicit attention, food or petting. The dog must walk properly on a leash, and not overreact to people, animals, bicyclists, or vehicles. The dog must enter and exit public buildings such as banks and hotels, and must ride on elevators. The dog must behave properly in a grocery store and not attempt to eat or sniff the merchandise. The dog must wait patiently while the handler speaks to other people, stands in a line, or shops for groceries.

The ideal age to start service-specific training is at two to three years of age, although obedience training and house training can begin in puppyhood. Before Service Dogs of New Mexico accepted Honeybits and me as a team in training, we had to pass a rigorous qualification process. As I go through the different decision criteria, I'll elaborate on how the selection process applies to Hearing Ear dogs in general and Honeybits in particular.

Does Size Matter?

Part of selecting a service dog requires the trainer—not the handler, but the trainer—to match the animal to the task. Most disabilities require work a tiny dog can't do: guide work, carrying work, bracing work, and such. A little Pomeranian, for example, cannot effectively guide a blind person, push a wheelchair, or serve as a PTSD dog who must make encroaching people physically back off by interposing his or her body between the handler and an oncoming person. It was only dumb luck that I happen to have the kind of disability little Honeybits could help with: I'm losing my hearing, not my sight or my balance. Although I've had surgery on both knees, I am not mobility impaired and I'm not yet at an age where other medical problems start to appear.

If you anticipate a need to brace against the dog to stand or to recover from a fall, obviously your dog must be strong enough to support you. If by chance you have more than one disability, or if you are approaching an age where a bad fall is a statistical likelihood, choose a larger dog.

In the dog training community, there are two schools of thought regarding whether smaller animals should be trained as alert dogs at all. Neither is necessarily "right" or "wrong" and both make very valid points.

Perspective #1: Strength, Reach, and the Ability to Make People Back Off

Because a service dog is a multi-year commitment, it makes sense to choose a larger animal as a Hearing Ear dog. A larger dog has strength, reach, and the ability to make other people back off should the need arise. These attributes, while not necessary for alert work in the home, make for a more versatile service animal if you ever develop the need for help with more than hearing related alerts.

It's important to consider not just the assistance work you need today, but what services you are likely to need within the next ten years. It is relatively easy to train a new behavior into a service dog you already have, provided he or she is physically able to do the work. But if that work involves bracing, opening doors, turning lights on and off, or pushing a wheelchair, a small dog simply cannot do the work for you.

Large dogs find it physically easy to climb stairs, hop up onto a chair or bed when necessary, or reach up to operate a light switch or a door handle. A small dog simply cannot reach things that are waist-height to a human. If the handler has difficulty reaching things or needs help with doors or lights in addition to alert behaviors, or if he or she expects to need that kind of help in the future, obviously the service dog has to be big enough to perform the work.

When you go out in public, a large dog is very visible. People instinctively make room for them. No Labrador retriever has ever been trampled or stepped on by someone who fails to notice him or her. This is important for the dog's safety. People also tend to not rush a large dog although they may try to pet the animal. People who cannot resist the miniature Dachshund in a service vest will back off from a German Shepherd or a Rottweiler. Early in an animal's training, before a service vest is an option, it's important to not accidentally train the animal to solicit or accept attention from strangers. A small dog who is a child magnet and who is petted and fussed over by everyone in sight may develop an attention-seeking habit that is difficult or impossible to train out. Furthermore, if you ever develop anxiety or PTSD, you will need a dog big enough to physically get between you and whoever is getting too close. A large dog is often a deterrent to people whose approach might be unwelcome, but a small dog just doesn't have the mass to perform that function.

Perspective #2: Life Span, Portability, and the Ability to Make People Come Closer

Because a service dog is a multi-year commitment, unless you anticipate a need for reaching or bracing related services it makes sense to choose a smaller animal as a Hearing Ear dog or alter dog. Smaller dogs live longer, are generally healthier, and have a longer working life than larger dogs. They travel far more easily especially in airplanes and vehicles, and they serve a very important social function because they bring people closer to you.

Given that training often can't begin until a dog is at least two years old, a large dog with an effective lifespan of ten years has at most six or seven good working years before old age sets in. A small dog such a Chihuahua, which can be expected to live eighteen years or more, will be able to work twice as long as a larger dog especially since Hearing Ear work is not physically strenuous. Since human beings live longer than dogs, a person who is born Deaf or hard of hearing might easily have several service dogs in his or her lifetime. A commitment to a large-dog strategy will cost twice as much in the long term, in training alone.

Small dogs require very little space. If you live in a small apartment or a nursing home, or if you travel or fly regularly, a small dog creates very little inconvenience. If you live in a dwelling with limited access to the outdoors—such as a high-rise apartment—finding toilet facilities when Fido has to go can be difficult. Most people keep fake grass, a square of sod, or puppy training pads on hand just in case, but large dogs create big puddles and big piles of waste that can leave a lingering odor especially if you have to leave the dog unattended. If you're like most Deaf or hard-of-hearing people, you will be working, going to school, running errands, or doing other things especially during the training period when your not-yet-official service dog can't accompany you. So your dog will have to take care of his or her toilet needs unsupervised, and you'll have to clean it up. Small dogs generate even less waste and mess than cats do.

Small dogs are non-threatening and cute. Provided they do not approach people or solicit attention, they create the impression that *you* are friendly and approachable. Everyone wants to pet the cute Yorkie or Silky Terrier. This can be a very good thing. Hearing loss is a very socially isolating condition, and if you're an introvert like me or if you have the noticeable speech deterioration that comes from using a cochlear implant, you may not be the sort of person to speak up and start conversations. There have been times in my life where several days at a time have gone by without me saying a word to another human being. If you've got a cute service dog, other people approach *you* and start interacting with you. If you live alone and don't have a support system, a cute dog can create a lifeline for you to the outside world.

If you haven't already guessed it, I'm a dedicated member of Team Tiny Dog. I've publicly expressed my support for small dogs in general, and Chihuahuas in particular, as Hearing Ear dogs. My Honeybits weighs only about five pounds, yet I rely on her as completely as I would if she were a Saint Bernard. Most Hearing Ear dogs I've met so far tend to be small, and their handlers assure me that the expense and logistics associated with smaller dogs, combined with their longer lifespans, more than justify whatever other tradeoffs there are.

Desirable Traits

To be an effective Hearing Ear dog, a candidate animal should have specific physical, mental, and emotional traits.

Age and Health

Two to three years of age is considered an ideal time to begin dog training. Puppies, as adorable as they are, are too emotionally immature and spastic to receive more than obedience and foundational training. They can and should be socialized and given obedience skills, yet there's no such thing as a service puppy.

A Hearing Ear dog should begin task specific training at less than four years of age (for a large dog) or less than five years of age (for a small one). If raised as a service dog from puppyhood, the dog generally receives general obedience training first and starts the disability-specific training at about age two. Since alert training takes much less time than guide dog training, it's possible to begin at a slightly later age especially if the dog has already received obedience and foundational training.

Health-wise, a Hearing Ear Dog must obviously have two functional ears. He or she should not be blind in either eye, and should be able-bodied without any missing limbs or chronic diseases. The dog should be able to move freely and to wear a leash with a harness, and should be able to walk distances of at least half a mile without tiring or suffering breathing difficulty. The dog should be able to breathe, eat, and drink normally and must be free of parasites or contagious diseases that could harm other animals. Most handlers provide their dogs with heartworm pills especially if they spend time outdoors.

Hearing Ear Dogs may be of any breed or gender, however a service dog must be spayed or neutered. This should ideally occur before training begins. Having birthed puppies in the past does not disqualify a bitch from Hearing Ear Dog work. Mutts are welcome because there is no breed or "pure-breed" requirement for Hearing Ear Dog work.

All service dogs, including Hearing Ear Dogs, are required to have all legally mandatory shots including the rabies vaccine. These shots must be kept current.

Intelligence and Trainability

A Hearing Ear Dog must be intelligent enough to master basic commands such as sit, down, and stay. If you are converting a pet into a service dog, he or she should already have passed the Canine Good Citizen (CGC) test administered by your country's Kennel Club. Inability to function on a leash, persistent straining at the collar, and excessive reaction to strange people or other dogs can sometimes be trained out, but the dog in question must be amenable to training.

Agility, tricks, dog parkour, and advanced obedience work requires intelligence. So does "nose work" or tracking. No service dog needs an actual title in such a sport, but the ability to learn basic commands is evidence of the kind of initiative and intelligence it takes to be an alert dog. If a dog has a history of being able to do tricks, advanced obedience, and other activities that require them to be out of the home and to learn new things, it's a mark in that dog's favor. Problem-solving and proactive play, in which a dog takes the initiative to get a human to play or to go for a walk, is evidence of the same kind of intelligence it takes to be an alert dog.

All service dogs must be housebroken and used to living with humans. Your dog should be used to living and sleeping indoors. You are welcome to crate-train the dog, and a separate bed and sleeping area for your service dog is always a good idea. But to do his or her work, a Hearing Ear Dog must have access to you even at night.

Temperament

All service dogs, without exception, must pass the Public Access Test. As part of the test, the dog must demonstrate appropriate, polite, and well socialized responses to people and animals. Whatever instincts the dog might have to bark, lunge, cower, chase, fixate, play, or solicit attention must be kept in check while the dog is working. The dog must not be excessively fearful, anxious, or aggressive. An extremely dominant or submissive attitude, with self-defense behaviors like growling or snapping, render a dog ineligible for service work. The service dog temperament is sometimes described as "mellow", "relaxed", or "even-tempered".

Willingness to obey, and to bond with the handler and be around him or her, is critical for any service animal. However the obedience should not take the very extreme form advocated by certain mainstream dog trainers who insist that you must always be the "pack leader", and that the dog should never do anything on his or her own initiative without your permission. That level of control simply isn't appropriate in a service animal who *must*, by definition, take the initiative sometimes to provide information you simply don't have. You might be the "master" or "mistress" to your pet or to your Schutzhund style protection dog, but with your service dog you're more of a partner. You definitely lead the dance, but there *are* times your dog will know better than you. If that wasn't the case, you wouldn't need an alert dog. Your dog should not attempt to dominate you, obviously, but must be capable of mutual communication. Sometimes there will be selective disobedience when your dog refuses to come along because he or she sees or hears something you can't, and is alerting you to something you need to know about.

An alert dog must be curious and aware of his or her surroundings. It's part of his or her job to look, turn, watch, listen, and respond to his or her environment. Your dog should not fixate on something like a smell, a ball, or a moving object to the point where you can't get or keep his or her attention. A dog who develops "tunnel vision" or who becomes fixated on things such as a ball, an object to chase, or a perceived threat can often get so wrapped up with the object of fixation that he or she cannot (not "will not" but "cannot") break his or her attention away to respond to a command. Such focus is desirable in a tracking animal or perhaps a herding animal, yet for service work it's a disadvantage. In fact, it can be downright dangerous.

Separation anxiety is not a disqualifying trait because the service dog and the human handler are not separated under normal circumstances.

All dogs have a prey drive and a chase instinct, however your dog should be able to understand and obey your commands even when distracted by a toy or a squirrel. A dog with an uncontrollable temper or prey drive cannot concentrate well enough on you or your needs to perform well as a service animal.

Your dog should be mellow enough to sit, stand, or lie down quietly at your feet while you sit or stand with the leash. A dog who startles or freaks out because of thunder, fireworks, or loud noises may have difficulty passing the Public Access Test.

A service dog must not display dominance or aggression toward people or animals, and must not lunge, growl, chase, or snap at other animals. But he or she should not be excessively fearful or submissive, because "self-defense" growling and snapping are also a form of aggression. The best dog for service dog is neither the stereotypical "alpha" animal who dominates the pack nor a very fearful, excitable one.

A service dog, regardless of size, should not display an aggressive or entitled mentality. The dreaded "small dog syndrome", in which a tiny animal tries to dominate or control his or her surroundings by biting, demonstrating aggression and territoriality, or deliberately misbehaving, is usually a result of lack of obedience training and socialization. Whereas large dogs are very likely to receive regular walks, deliberate training, and structured obedience classes, small dogs are often let loose to run wild in a house or yard and denied even the most basic obedience training. The same behavior that would be horrifying in a Saint Bernard or a Great Dane is described as "funny" or "cute" when a Pomeranian or Chihuahua does it. Therefore, small dogs often go without the patient correction or training that would allow them to develop good, non-destructive habits. That, sadly, renders the dog ineligible for service training of any kind.

All service dogs must recover quickly from startling or stressful situations once the source of the stress is removed. Being barked at by a larger dog, or being in a crowded room with many people, should not cause the dog to melt down. If your dog responds to short-term stress by turning into a furry puddle, so that you have to carry him or her out of a stressful situation, or if your dog remains on edge minutes or hours after the danger has passed, this dog cannot do service work. You definitely need for your dog to alert you to danger, but a dog that *keeps* alerting after the danger has passed will not serve you well.

"Not being able to recover and calm down," says Jennifer Hunt, an owner and professional trainer at Duke City Dog Academy, "is a trait that cannot be trained out. There's a lot that can be done to desensitize a dog to noises or situations that might be frightening or overwhelming, but if the dog stays tense or gradually becomes more nervous that's more likely to be an expression of a genetic trait."

Dogs who are played with as puppies and given obedience classes and introduction to other animals tend to be better behaved compared to dogs who don't have the opportunity. They are far more likely to show the calm, patient, non-aggressive temperament needed to succeed as service dogs. One key factor in helping to guarantee that a pup grows into service dog material is to ensure that he or she is exposed to children and toddlers. In this area, small dogs tend to be underserved by the rescue community and the dog owning community, because many people believe that children should *never* be around small dogs. A small dog who is denied exposure to toddlers never learns that they are only playing and that a baby lacks enough mass or strength to do serious damage even intentionally.

Socialization

A service dog needs to be people-oriented and not dog-oriented. During the imprinting period, the puppy should have had contact with people of all different shapes and sizes. It is not necessary for your service dog to be comfortable with other dogs or with cats, provided there's no aggression or chasing. Indeed, a certain aloofness and lack of desire to play with strange dogs is an asset in service dog work.

According to Bennie Jean Muliere, founder of Service Dogs of New Mexico, many service dog training organizations insist on breeding and raising their own dogs from puppyhood to ensure that the animals they provide to clients are well socialized, housebroken, and generally healthy. There's an advantage to this approach: the animal's entire medical and behavioral history is known, and the animal's environment is controlled to ensure that he or she is exposed to different kinds of animals, people, and situations in a reasonable way so that no undue fear or chase responses develop. However, for reasons related to speed and the ability to serve a larger number of people who need service dogs, some training organizations make use of owner surrenders, foster animals, or dogs that the clients find themselves. These dogs still have to be screened for other desirable traits, but the advantage to training clients who already have their prospective service dog is that the dog is already well bonded to the handler.

Disqualifying Traits

There are a few traits that disqualify an animal from service work. They include physical impairments that make it impossible for an animal to continue working and behavioral problems that make it inadvisable to even start the training process. A reputable trainer will not willingly put time or effort into a physically, mentally, or emotionally unfit animal with the goal of turning him or her into a service dog. It's unethical to waste a customer's time or money. Before the customer sinks thousands of hours (and dollars!) into training, he or she deserves at least reasonable certainty that the training process will produce an animal capable of passing the Public Access Test.

I ought to note that an animal who is unsuitable for service work can still be a good pet. The services of a professional animal trainer can help a fearful dog learn trust, and can take the edge off an assertive animal. However, service dogs are permitted everywhere, including where pets are not allowed and where ordinary people would not expect dogs to be. Compared to a pet, a service dog's duties are more physically strenuous and require far more intelligence, concentration, and emotional balance.

There are three reasons why disqualifying traits render an animal unsuitable for service work. First, the trait may render the animal physically incapable of performing his or her tasks. For example, a dog with no hearing cannot alert a Deaf person to noise, because the dog cannot respond to what he or she can't hear. Likewise, a dog who cannot climb stairs due to hip dysplasia cannot jump or climb onto the bed to awaken his or her sleeping handler when the fire alarm is sounding and the house is on fire.

A trait may be disqualifying if it puts the animal at risk during the performance of a task. My Honeybits could never be qualified as a mobility assistance dog because if anyone tried to brace against her to climb into a wheelchair, she would be injured. Since alert dogs don't need to brace, small size is not a disqualifying trait for Hearing Ear dogs, although it is for mobility assistance dogs. An example of a disqualifying trait for a Hearing Ear dog would be chronic patellar luxation, which tends to occur in small dog breeds. If a Hearing Ear dog cannot walk any significant distance without dislocating his or her own knee, service work is simply too risky.

The third way a trait may be disqualifying is if it puts other people, or their animals, or their property, at risk. You have the right to bring a service dog with you everywhere you go (with a few exceptions such as people's homes and sterile environments such as operating rooms or commercial food preparation areas).

You are liable, legally and financially, for any damage your service dog does. If your service dog injures someone by biting or jumping up, if he or she hurts or kills a smaller dog who is running about off-leash, or if there's significant damage to property, the person you hurt has the right to sue for damages especially if no reasonable person would have been aware of the danger. Service dogs are generally considered to be "safe". So if a service dog bites someone, especially in a confined space, it makes headlines.

In the United States, and many other countries also, there are two kinds of liability: civil liability (where the person you hurt files suit against you to make you pay for the damage you cause), and criminal liability (where the city, state, county, or nation charges you with a crime for which you may be fined or imprisoned). If your dog harms someone, you will be found guilty of criminal negligence if the prosecution can show that you knew, or had reason to know, that you were putting other people at risk by bringing an aggressive animal into their presence. A dog with a history of biting or aggression to people or animals is not an animal you want to expose to the public especially in a confined space like an elevator or an airplane.

Physically Unfit Dogs

A dog who is deaf, blind, or otherwise unable to respond to his or her environment cannot function as a service dog. Nor can an animal who is too old, obese, or sick to walk or to perform the functions of his or her service work. A Hearing Ear Dog who cannot hear well enough to locate the source of a sound, who cannot see well enough to respond to your hand signal, or who cannot hop up onto the couch or your bed to wake you up when the fire alarm is sounding is unable to perform a critical function of his or her work.

Minor traits that would be "disqualifications" or "serious faults" in a dog show, such as a tail shape that does not conform to the breed standard or a slight overbite or underbite that does not interfere with eating, are not disqualifications from a service dog perspective provided the dog is young, fit, and in excellent health. Honeybits, for example, has an underbite and her front legs turn out at the elbows in a way that wouldn't go over well in a show ring. But her teeth are excellent and the underbite doesn't prevent her from eating. The elbow issue is purely cosmetic, and after two years of puppy parkour, her legs are strong and her knees are likely to remain sound. Her ability to do her work doesn't depend on her appearance.

No reputable trainer will knowingly provide service dog training to an animal that is elderly or that suffers from a genetic problem such as hip dysplasia or uncorrected chronic patellar luxation. Diseases such as canine diabetes or kidney problems can render a dog ineligible to begin training, although many handlers continue to employ working dogs who develop illnesses. At some point, elderly and sick dogs do have to retire. A working dog is supposed to be an asset whose presence enhances your life, not a liability whose presence encumbers you.

Even the best service dogs eventually age and have to retire, although a Hearing Ear Dog whose work is performed mostly in the home can generally continue doing it longer than most. But a dog that becomes incontinent cannot be taken into a store or restaurant. Once his or her bladder or bowel control becomes flaky, he or she must be retired from public access.

When a service dog becomes too old or sick to work in his or her normal capacity, he or she usually lives out the rest of his or her natural life as an honored member of the handler's family, receiving appropriate food, exercise, and veterinary care. An injured, blind, or sickly dog *can* be an outstanding pet. Just look at all the videos of three-legged dogs, one-eyed dogs, or other animals who are well loved by their families. But a working dog with a disability isn't quite the same as a human who has one. The dog's job can seldom be altered to adapt for the dog's disability to allow the dog to remain "employed". You, for example, will be relying on your dog to do your hearing for you. This means that you and the dog can't *both* be deaf at the same time. Many dogs lose their hearing in old age, and if that happens to your Hearing Ear Dog, it's time to set aside the vest.

Lack of Housebreaking

A dog that cannot be trained to urinate and defecate in appropriate places is a poor choice for a service dog. Former "puppy mill" dogs or animals sold from pet stores often lose the natural instinct to not urinate or defecate near their food or in the den. They can be extremely hard to housebreak, and often cannot be taken out in public. The same goes for dogs that "mark" or spray urine regularly. An animal that marks the carpet and the children's toys in your home will also mark the carpet in a store or an airplane.

Destructiveness is another mark of a dog that is poorly housebroken. A properly housebroken adult dog who is not a teething puppy can be allowed the run of your house overnight or while you are at work. You will awaken or return to find that the dog has not chewed up the carpet or flooring, scratched holes in the wall, or destroyed your shoes or clothing. A dog who destroys your belongings or carpet will destroy other people's as well. Honeybits, for example, has access to my entire home. As long as I keep truly tempting items like pens and tissue paper out of reach, she can be trusted in any corner of my house.

Suppose for a moment that, against all odds, you manage to get a dog through the Public Access Test despite his or her habit of chewing up linoleum or tearing up carpet. Congratulations: you've earned your ID card and a vest for your pooch. You now have the right of access into even the swankiest hotel, and the law requires landlords to rent to you without charging a pet fee or otherwise protecting themselves against damage done by your dog. So, you rent a hotel room for the night when you're traveling for business, or you sign a lease for an apartment. Sooner or later, though, you're going to have to leave your dog unattended while you sleep, or use the restroom, or walk to the mailbox. You may have scheduled surgery that keeps you in the hospital for a little while, and although you've arranged to have someone check on your dog you aren't there in person. So, for whatever reason, there's a delay of some kind that results in you taking your eyes off the dog. You awaken or return to a scene out of John Grogan's *Marley & Me: Life and Love with the World's Worst Dog.*

Even a small animal can cause thousands of dollars' worth of destruction. Urine soaks through carpet and can be absorbed in the padding underneath it. It is absorbed by wooden baseboards and by drywall. Once that happens, the only practical repair is to rip out the contaminated part and replace it. Although the law forbids landlords to charge you extra rent, you *are* legally and financially liable for any damage your service dog happens to do. This might include damage to flooring, walls, cabinetry, fences, or landscaping.

The Grogans owned the house that Marley destroyed, so they had the option of renovating when and if they chose to do so. Your landlord, if you rent, will not be so understanding and may demand that you repair damages immediately. If you're staying in a hotel or motel, you're liable for every knocked-over lamp or weird-smelling spot on the carpet. The fact that you did not personally cause the damage is irrelevant. Your dog, your teenager, or your party guests might do any number of thing to the property you rent, but *you* are the one with your name on the dotted line.

Aggression

Aggression toward people and other animals is a disqualifying trait because it cannot reliably be trained out. Any dog who has bitten a person or another animal (except in self-defense or in defense of a family member) is too aggressive for service work. One of the reasons it's important to know an animal's history is because sometimes aggressive behavior doesn't become obvious until an animal has been put in a situation that brings it out. A dog who is food-aggressive, for example, may react poorly to being told to leave or drop edible-smelling items on the ground. A dog who has bad memories related to people who, for example, smoke cigarettes or happen to be male, will tend to be protective and aggressive out of a sense of self preservation.

Human beings, when placed in a bad or unnatural situation, often develop unusual survival strategies. These strategies, if they become habitual, can turn into a maladaptive behavior that doesn't work very well in normal life. Animals who have been abused or neglected do the same. An animal who is underfed, the way performing animals often are, will develop aggressive behaviors related to food or to avoiding punishment. Dogs who are rescued from unscrupulous "puppy mill" breeders or dog fighting rings are often unable to breed, eat, mate, or interact normally with other dogs. But unlike humans, who can sometimes unlearn the bad and maladaptive behaviors in order to enjoy a positive and fulfilling life, most animals have difficulty getting beyond their earliest conditioning and imprinting. Cognitive behavioral training unfortunately doesn't work as well on them as it does on us. So aggression, once developed, is extremely difficult to "train out".

There are rescue dogs who are advertised as "having to be the only pets in the house". This is a code phrase that means they physically harm other animals and that they cannot be trusted around cats, small animals, or children. Such animals, while they are still worthy of respect and love, simply cannot become service animals. The same goes for obsessively dominant animals.

A dog that has been trained to fight or to perform protection ("Schutzhund") work cannot be a service animal. Retired military or police dogs generally become the pets of their former handlers, and are never repurposed to service dog work.

Excessive Territoriality

A dog that barks aggressively at strangers who walk by the house or yard, who mounts the legs of visitors to your home, or who "marks" by urinating on every available surface, may be a little too territorial to be a good service animal. Although most of your Hearing Ear Dog's work will be done in the home, you must also be able to welcome plumbers, electricians, emergency medical workers, and relatives.

Most mammals have a territorial instinct of some kind: they know where their home is. Humans have been exploiting the den instincts of their watchdogs and guard dogs since before the earliest recorded history. But there's such a thing as too much of a territorial instinct, because a very territorial animal has an exaggerated perception of threat. This exaggerated perception may cause the animal to behave aggressively or defensively when no real threat exists.

A good Hearing Ear Dog will inform you when there's someone at the door, and then *allow you to respond to the visitor in the way you believe is appropriate*. An overly territorial dog will take it upon himself or herself to scare away a perceived intruder or to assert dominance once the newcomer arrives.

In most of your interactions with your dog, you must be the "alpha" partner. That doesn't mean that you bully or dominate your dog—it simply means that you are the default decision maker. Your dog should follow your instructions and your leadership. Only in rare occasions will a service dog selectively disobey, stopping you mid-walk to alert you to someone approaching rapidly from behind, or refusing to walk with you into a busy intersection or around a blind corner when a person is waiting on the other side with bad intentions. Selective disobedience is a very sophisticated behavior that only the most intelligent dogs display. It is not the same as the mindless disobedience that occurs when a dog becomes fixated on an activity or an object and simply ignores your attempts to make a forbidden activity stop.

A dog who mounts people's legs or who barks mindlessly when left alone in someone's backyard all day is simply disobedient. A dog who disobeys because the dog thinks he or she knows best, who is *not* actually in a position to know best, simply can't be trained to serve you. There are situations in which your service dog must selectively disobey, when he or she sees or hears a threat that you can't. But this is a radically different behavior from behaving badly simply because the dog has some maladaptive behaviors or thinks he or she is the boss.

Fearfulness

An animal who displays extreme submissiveness and fearfulness toward people or toward other animals cannot pass the Public Access Test. Fearful dogs may bite out of a perceived need for self-defense. This is not a problem that is easily corrected.

Most animals will lash out if they're in pain, and if you pick up an animal who has just been injured or who is recovering from surgery and is not quite conscious, you may be bitten. It's an instinctive response and not something that's under the animal's conscious control. Human beings who are coming out of general anesthesia after a major surgery also sometimes say and do things that are uncharacteristic of them, simply because they're chemically impaired. They don't even remember it afterwards. But that's an instinctive response that is very different from ongoing fearfulness and excessively submissive behavior.

Animals mostly don't like to be loomed over or grabbed by strangers. They're not Tokyo, and you're not Godzilla. So if you come at them as though you are, the obvious solution for the dog is to back away and to give you space. If you persist, the dog will become even more agitated because you're behaving rudely and failing to respect his or her body language. The same thing happens if poorly socialized dogs insist on pressing forward, sniffing, and ignoring the canine equivalent of the word "no". This kind of backing off is not fearfulness: it's a very reasonable response to being stalked or surrounded by people who don't back off when you ask them to.

If you were in an unfamiliar space and a very large and out of control person was trying to grab you or touch your body after you'd backed away and asked him or her to stop, you'd get upset too. What would happen next depends on your own personality and social skills. You might raise your voice, you might call for help, you might run away, or you might deliver a well-placed uppercut. It's unreasonable to expect a higher standard of conduct from our dogs than we do from ourselves. But response to the bad or inappropriate behaviors of others is not the same as fearfulness.

A fearful dog is afraid of *all* or perhaps *most* people or dogs. He or she doesn't seek out or accept affection from anybody and cannot walk by a well-behaved specimen of the species without barking, lunging, or trying to get away. Excessive reactivity to people or to other dogs is often due to poor socialization or lack of exposure. Mild reactivity is correctable, but if your dog is stressed by the presence of other human beings and other dogs, he or she can't help you when out in public.

Anxious or Reactive Behavior

An animal who is tense and on edge might provide a great alert, but he or she cannot be brought out in public. One of the things a service dog must do is return to a lower level of emotional arousal after an unusual or scary situation. A dog who holds onto his or her fear and who gradually becomes more tense and reactive while under stress has difficulty adapting to new environments, which by definition are stressful.

A reactive dog is one who overreacts to people, other animals, or other stimulus. The word "reactive" should not be confused with the word "responsive". For an alert dog of any type, you want an animal who is basically curious and interested in his or her surroundings. You want one who responds to what he or she sees and hears. The kind of dog who curls up at your feet and instantly goes to sleep when you sit down may not be alert enough to wake up when there's a siren or a loud noise. But you do not want the dog to *overreact* by barking, showing aggression, soliciting attention, or cowering in fear.

Yappiness

You and I will obviously never be bothered by a dog who yaps its head off for no good reason, who barks at every person who walks by the house or yard, or who bays randomly several times a day or who howls and barks continually when left alone. Such dogs exist, but they don't form part of our world. Even if they are baying at the top of their lungs, we are blissfully unaware of the fact. We can't hear them. But everyone else can, and how your dog behaves will influence how the rest of the world reacts to you.

When I say that Honeybits isn't yappy, I'm not relying solely on my own perception or experience. That would be disingenuous at best. I have objective confirmation of the fact that although she frequently vocalizes with squeaks, grunts, or wa-wa sounds, she rarely barks.

Dogs raised from puppyhood in Deaf of hard-of-hearing households seldom bark. There's no point, and they learn early that it isn't an effective attention-getting behavior. Sooner or later, I predict that Deaf people will realize that they have an excellent and unique business opportunity: their homes are an ideal place to raise puppies for service work of all kinds. They can provide basic housebreaking and obedience training until he or she is old enough to take on more specialized tasks, then turn them over to whatever charity matches the dogs with their handlers. Dogs raised in such an environment grow up unaware that they can get attention by barking or vocalizing. A dog who learns early to get your attention by tapping you, nosing you, rubbing against you, or entering your line of sight will never become yappy.

We hard-of-hearing people must avoid the temptation to pat ourselves on the back for raising non-yappy dogs. The fact our dogs respond to the environment, stimulus, or reinforcement we provide them, and the fact that we tend to reinforce attention-seeking behaviors other than barking, do not constitute moral superiority on our part. Plenty of dogs in hard-of-hearing households find other ways to be cheeky.

Yappiness is contagious. A dog who seldom barks will often "learn" to do it if he or she spends significant time around a dog who has learned that barking and yapping will eventually draw the owner's attention. Once yappiness sets in, the only way to correct it is to rigorously fail to respond to barking while monitoring the dog and proactively rewarding the slightest alternate behavior that isn't a bark. Ignoring the dog completely while he or she is barking is a bad idea because dogs do periodically try other strategies when the first one doesn't work. If you ignore the dog completely while the dog is barking for attention, you will miss the other things they do: the point, the rolling over, the gentle tap with the paw or the nudge with the nose. That's the behavior you must acknowledge and reward. Once the dog learns how to get the attention he or she wants, he or she will use the strategy in preference to others.

There's such a thing as incorrigible barking. A dog fostered in a Deaf or hard-of-hearing household who persists in barking as a primary mode of communication, who doesn't figure out in a matter of hours or days that barking isn't the solution to any problem in particular, is either dim-witted or too set in his or her ways to find reasons to change. Continuing to display the one behavior guaranteed to not be an effective alert, if the residents of the house are attempting to interact and to mark the attention-getting behaviors they want, disqualifies the dog for sheer stupidity if for nothing else.

A Competing Bond

One of the last disqualifying traits, and a very common one in households where a pet is being considered for service dog training, is the presence of a strong emotional bond with one or more people besides the dog's future handler. A dog who bonds with one person can and will bond with a second one if the first owner dies or if the dog is rehomed. But in such cases, the formation of the new bond only becomes possible because the first bond is completely extinguished.

Family pets tend to bond with everyone in a household to some extent or another. Cats and some breeds of dogs such as Chihuahuas tend to have a favorite person, but part of the process of raising a dog in a family requires that the dog accept instruction or correction from *all* the family members. This is sometimes expressed in "pack leader" terminology, but more often it represents a social bond between the family member and the dog.

A service dog's primary bond has to be with his or her handler. If the dog has a favorite person who for some reason is *not* the handler, there's going to be a problem because the dog will prefer his or her favorite person and seek out that person's company instead of staying close to the person who needs the service dog.

My Honeybits was originally supposed to be an emotional support animal for my teenaged daughter, whom I'd adopted a few months before. My daughter carried the puppy around for a couple weeks, and everything seemed to be going well because the dog adored my daughter. Then the novelty wore off and my kid lost all interest in the dog. The tiny pup, sensing something was badly wrong, appealed to the only other large, warm-blooded object in sight: me. Had that not occurred, Honeybits would not have been a suitable service animal for me.

I never set out to deliberately alienate Honeybits from my daughter. It happened naturally, one pup-snuggle at a time, until eventually the dog turned to me instead of to my daughter. She bonded well enough with me to pass all her obedience classes at Camp Bow Wow, where she earned her CGC at the age of sixteen months. I used the clicker based training to develop Honeybits's door recognition behaviors, and we were accepted by Service Dogs of New Mexico before she was even two years old. Her training went well—she averaged one new behavior per lesson—and she is an outstanding ambassador for Hearing Ear dogs in general, and Chihuahuas in particular.

Service Dogs of New Mexico approved Honeybits to train with me because she had all the qualifying traits and none of the disqualifying ones. The plan worked because Honeybits was bonded with *me*. My daughter had moved out by that point, but had she been present and strongly bonded with Honeybits the training may have failed. It's OK for a service dog to recognize familiar people and to prefer some over others, but his or her primary bond *must* be with the handler.

The presence of competing bonds is one of the reasons why many household pets aren't able to transition to service work. If one family member has a disability or needs help but the dog prefers to spend time around a different family member, the differently abled person may not be able to successfully train the dog. Sometimes the family members themselves can unwittingly interfere with training. From the moment service training begins, the person primarily responsible for feeding and walking the dog must be the handler. No other person should sleep with the dog, and if the family is watching TV together the dog should be at the feet or in the lap of the handler, not being snuggled by a different family member. When a dog is a "family" pet, the old habits are hard to break, and unless the animal's primary bond is *already* with the hard-of-hearing person, it's going to be almost impossible to redirect.

Chapter 7: Where to Get the Dog

At first glance, it seems like a no-brainer: if there are tens of thousands of physically capable young dogs in shelters and also tens of thousands of people who need service animals, wouldn't it make sense to snap up the shelter dogs and start training them? Well... the answer turns out to be no.

The idea of using shelter dogs for service dog work is kind of like the theoretical notion of using a bunch of undeveloped land to provide housing for the homeless. It looks good on paper, but there are reasons *why* most undeveloped land remains undeveloped. Lack of water, unstable geology, and commuting distance all affect the price of land and a developer's desire to invest in it. Unless the odds are high that the housing built will match the needs of the people for whom it is intended, no developer will risk building. A few empty apartments eat up all the potential profit from the venture, and if the *majority* of the apartments can't meet the existing housing codes, they simply can't be sold and are therefore not worthwhile to train. It's the same with service animals. Unless the odds are high that the dog can be trained to pass the Public Access Test and to conduct himself or herself well with a handler who has disabilities, it's unfair to both the dog and the handler to begin the training process or to allow a bond to form.

In the orientation provided to all prospective service dog handlers by Service Dogs of New Mexico (SDNM), Executive Director Bennie Muliere shares information about how service dogs are recruited and trained. Unlike many organizations that breed and raise their dogs from puppyhood, SDNM *will* accept a qualified adult dog for training provided he or she has all the desirable traits, none of the disqualifying traits, and the physical attributes necessary to do the work. A few of us handlers do end up finding or bringing suitable dogs, but most of SDNM's dogs are either owner surrenders or dogs who have been fostered for several months.

"We never accept a trainee dog directly from a shelter," says Ms. Muliere. "We tried it several times, early on, but I can count our successes on the fingers of one hand and have fingers left over. There were far, far more failures. And every dog who enters training, who bonds to a handler, and who fails to become a qualified service dog by learning the appropriate disability service behaviors and passing the Public Access test creates a huge emotional and financial burden. Every month invested in training an animal is a month the handler has to go without a trained and qualified dog."

Training is expensive. Whether the cost is borne by the handler or by some charity or grant dedicated to providing animals to a specific category of people with disabilities, nobody likes wasting money. After enough failures, or after an incident in which a trained and qualified service dog loses his or her temper and bites someone, a trainer loses credibility. Even a grant-giving organization wants to ensure that its money is making a difference in the lives of people with disabilities and not just paying people to play with puppies.

It takes months, or sometimes years, to fully train a service dog. How long it takes depends on the temperament of the dog and the complexity of the service. A Seeing Eye dog for a blind person takes years to train. In comparison, a Hearing Ear dog can sometimes be trained in as little as six to eight months. The time investment is still enormous. When the handlers are training their own dogs they routinely work with the animals every day, spending an hour or more per day in training. Providing food and medical care to an animal in training is not cheap or free, and professional trainers do charge fees. Even if these fees are covered by a charitable grant, the handler's time and emotional investment is significant.

Why Shelter Dogs Fail

Many dogs end up in a shelter because they are badly socialized, untrained, and therefore aggressive, destructive, or otherwise badly behaved. Some have been abused or neglected. Eventually the dog begins to act out to the point where he or she is unwelcome. He or she might compulsively urinate on carpet, bite someone, kill livestock, or seriously injure another pet. For whatever reason, the dog owner decides to give up. That doesn't mean the owner hates the dog. Frequently the owner cares for the dog and wants to give him or her a good chance to succeed in a new home. So instead of telling the truth about the behavior problem, the owner lies. He or she makes up some nonsense about having to move or developing an allergy.

Very few people surrender or rehome their animals on a whim. They generally love their dogs and make at least some attempt to correct unwanted behaviors, yet if their approach is inconsistent or if they're unable to correct the problem, it often takes months or years before they give up. By this time the unwanted behavior has often become entrenched.

People seldom acknowledge their own role in creating a problem. They like to think of themselves as "good" people and "good" dog owners, so it's easier to believe that the *dog* is bad. Most of the "bad dog" behavior in *Marley and Me* was a puppy's response to an environment that wasn't suited to teach him good behavior. Of course, blaming the dog won't get the animal accepted into the shelter or adopted out to another family, and a "good" dog owner who has to surrender a pet obviously tries to give the dog the best possible chance for a new life. Therefore, to keep their self-images intact and to preserve their notion that they are "good", many people who surrender their animals blow a lot of smoke. They come up with a very good reason why they are giving the dog up, in a way that doesn't assign blame to the dogs or to themselves.

Sometimes the lies people tell when surrendering their animals have a grain of truth in them. A person who is "moving to another apartment where dogs aren't allowed" might indeed be moving. Their destination may indeed be a dog-free zone. But there are almost always apartments that accept pets, even if the owner has to make do with fewer rooms or amenities because of the bigger pet deposit. A person who is truly committed to his or her animal will accept a lower standard of living to keep a creature he or she regards as a family member. The person with the "moving" excuse is far more likely to have been evicted due to problems related to the dog, and the solution—for the person, at least—is to use the move as an excuse to get rid of the animal. The person may have been evicted due to ongoing noise complaints because the dog will not stop barking or howling, or because of failure to repair extreme damage done by a dog who is not housebroken. The root cause of the problem—a dog who has developed bad habits due to being left alone and given insufficient training and exercise—conveniently gets ignored. The person who created the problem by not interacting enough with the dog and by not meeting the dog's needs gets off scot-free, and the "problem animal" is passed on to someone else. Sometimes the new home will work out beautifully simply because it doesn't contain whatever triggered the "problem" behavior. A dog with separation anxiety does fine in a home where he or she isn't left alone. A dog who dislikes cats does fine in a home that has none. That works out well if the dog is going to be a pet, because the home can be adapted to the animal. It doesn't work so well for service dog, because public space can't adapt to the individual.

A family that is giving up a "dog who doesn't get along with the other pets" may understate the seriousness of the problem. They have usually ignored aggression or failed to provide training or correction until the dog has seriously injured or killed another animal. The cute puppy who is "too much to handle" may have been taken from his or her mother too early before being taught proper bite control. The animal who has been tormented and abused by badly behaved children or members of the household will generally have an extreme aversion to anyone who resembles his or her abuser. Some people think it's fun or practical to teach their dog protection-type or attack behaviors, and we've all heard about dog fighting rings and puppy mills. But in order to protect the abuser, the puppy mill, or whatever human being created the problem, the truth must be swept under the rug.

Nobody ever surrenders an animal because he or she is too well housebroken, quiet, friendly, well behaved, cute, healthy, affordable, well socialized, and obedient. Even when a dog owner dies, an outstanding dog generally has enough people in the community who love him or her to ensure that Fido gets a good home, especially if the owner leaves an insurance policy or property to go along with the dog.

If I dropped dead tomorrow, for example, there is a long line of people who want Honeybits, many of whom can hear perfectly well. My precious little "Wawa" will never see the inside of an animal shelter. Too many people know her, love her, and are looking out for her. Plus, there's a clause in my will that sets aside a very decent chunk of change and a list of specific individuals who have offered to take her.

Upon arriving at a shelter, which is a very stressful and unnatural environment, dogs generally receive some kind of temperament test to determine whether the animal is too violent or too dangerous to be adopted out. Most dogs who aren't out of their minds with fear based aggression can pass this test. But that doesn't mean they are free of digging, chewing, or peeing problems. No animal shelter is capable of performing an exhaustive test to determine what an animal's real problems are, how they came about, or whether they can be corrected. So, many animal shelters allow dogs with severe behavioral problems to be adopted out simply because they aren't aware the problems exist. They often haven't been told about the problems, they obviously can't read the minds of the people who are surrendering animals, and if the animal in question is picked up as a stray there's absolutely no way to know his or her history.

Even when an animal in a rescue environment displays behavioral problems, there's a certain amount of optimistic self-delusion in the animal rescue and sheltering community. People truly want to believe that there's no such thing as a "bad" dog or one who cannot go on to live a healthy and happy life in the right environment. But even the famous Cesar Milan sometimes admits defeat when there's an animal so compulsively dominant by nature, or so twisted by abuse, that he or she simply cannot be socialized well enough to be a pet, much less a very reliable and trustworthy service animal.

A shelter animal can sometimes be rehabilitated as a pet, if the right home can be found to accommodate the animal's special needs. But if the animal's behavior is not controllable outside the home he or she cannot do service dog work. There are a very few shelter animals who do *not* have significant behavioral problems that can eventually be discovered after spending a few weeks or months with the dog. But separating the proverbial wheat from the chaff requires an enormous amount of time and resources that would be better spent on a dog who stands a high chance of completing the Public Access Test.

Like it or not, dogs have specific times in their lives when they are biologically disposed to imprint on human beings, to accept different kinds of people or animals without fear or aggression, and to learn to be out in different situations without melting down emotionally. A dog who isn't socialized as a puppy *can* be taught to tolerate human contact, but he or she will generally not seek out humans for companionship and may not be able to bond with a handler.

It's said that you can't teach an old dog new tricks. That adage isn't true, but dogs who have established habits are generally harder to train than dogs who haven't. Most shelter dogs have at least one or two bad habits that make them unsuitable for service work.

Foster Dogs Succeed

Nearly all the rescue dogs trained as service animals by Service Dogs of New Mexico are foster dogs. Foster dogs have an extremely good track record. A shelter dog can become a foster dog, if he or she is placed in a home environment with someone who has a good track record with the type of dog in question.

A foster based rescue is different from an animal shelter. Foster based rescue organizations sometimes draw their animals out of shelters and serve as more of a step-down form of care for animals that need better socialization or remedial training before they can be placed as pets (or, in your case, a service animal).

In a foster rescue, the dog is kept for a few weeks, or even months, by a family dedicated to finding out what makes the dog tick. The foster family keeps track of everything: how the dog behaves around kids, whether the animal is food-aggressive, and whether basic obedience commands have been learned. For this reason, people who genuinely *are* forced to give up a perfectly good and loyal animal due to some disaster generally take the time to find the best possible placement for him or her. They don't simply turn the animal loose on a deserted road, advertise the dog on the Internet, or hand him or her over to a 72-hour animal shelter. They try first to re-home the animal with someone they know, and if that doesn't work, they look for a foster based rescue.

Many foster-based rescue societies are dedicated to a specific breed or type of dog. Some emphasize lap dogs; others focus on working dog breeds. The charity pays the medical and food related expenses for the dog, but he or she is placed into a family that focuses on doing whatever it takes to care for him or her until a permanent adoption becomes available. During this time, the family puts the dog through his or her paces to find out what the animal is like and what kind of home would be best.

A dog who has been fostered for a few months has generally been exposed to lots of different kinds of people and animals. The foster family has spent lots of time observing the dog, walking on a leash, taking the animal to the vet, and interacting in a variety of circumstances. Sometimes they will provide training or rehabilitative work, and during the course of this work they will notice if the dog has any fixations, phobias, or medical problems that might restrict the type of home he or she may later live in. This process screens out dogs who are not good candidates for service training. A dog who has lived peacefully in a foster home has plenty of opportunity to display the desirable service dog traits, and to not display the disqualifying traits.

A foster animal who is housebroken, who has mastered basic obedience commands, and who interacts appropriately with people and animals might be a great candidate as a service dog trainee, *if* the dog's background is known and *if* the animal is free of any other disqualifying characteristics. An experienced trainer who fosters the dog a few months can generally assess his or her odds of success: I recently met a beautiful Australian Cattle Dog cross who, having been fostered by a professional trainer for six months, had already received his foundational obedience training. When he was matched with a handler, the training went very well and proceeded rapidly. This is a radically different situation compared to a dog found at a shelter who has received no socialization, housebreaking, or training.

Don't get me wrong: a shelter dog can *become* a foster dog, and can proceed from there to service dog training. Many foster based rescues draw their animals from shelters. Such dogs often receive basic obedience training and housebreaking from their foster families, and this sets the dog up to bond with his or her handler and to achieve success as a service animal assuming he or she doesn't have any disqualifying traits. But going directly from the shelter into service dog training is a recipe for disaster for all but the luckiest pairs.

Many of the organizations involved with service dog training are charitable ventures. But incorporating as a not-for-profit organization or obtaining tax exempt status doesn't protect you from being judged based on your results. Reputation counts, and your success rate is part of your reputation. If you consistently graduate dogs who act out in public, the quality of the dogs you graduate reflects on you. Nobody who reads a news article about one of your dogs who bites someone will care whether the dog in question had a traumatic background. As a handler, or as a trainer, your reputation will depend on the dog you train. If a dog you train ends up in the news for biting someone, your professional reputation will suffer. Donors, grant-giving charities, and people who are in a position to pay for your services may stop doing it.

As I said in my book *Sustainable Non-Profit Management*, being a charity or a not-for-profit corporation won't protect you from the legal consequences of what you do. If you train and endorse a dog who is aggressive, reactive, or maladjusted you will be just as liable as you would be if you were a private business. You will be held to the same standards as anybody else. If you live in a state where dog trainers are licensed or authorized to conduct the Public Access Test or to supervise service dog training, your authority to do this can and will be revoked if you don't maintain high standards.

Puppies Can Take a While

We *all* love puppies: precious, floppy-eared bundles of warmth who wiggle appealingly when we pick them up and who gaze soulfully up at us. But a puppy is also an incredible amount of work. Puppies chew things, pee and poop in inappropriate places, and sometimes have trouble moderating their bite force. They race around the house at top speed, they get into everything, and they display what I affectionately call "puppy spaz". They require training to ensure that they do not stare at other dogs or display inappropriate manners. They also need much more regular meals and trips to an appropriate potty site.

I raised Honeybits from puppyhood, but for three solid months I had to leave work at lunchtime and drive across town to feed her, potty her, and play with her. It was very disruptive to my work schedule. The general rule is that a dog can control his or her bladder or bowels for one hour per month of life. If you're away at work, or if nobody is home to care for the puppy, it's very difficult to do a good job of it solo. Puppy training and socialization classes are available once the little dog has all of his or her shots, yet the prime time to socialize a puppy is in the first few *weeks* of life. Furthermore, there are several rounds of shots involved. It wasn't until Honeybits was about nine months old that I started serious obedience training with her, and her late start with dog socialization set her back.

During a puppy's first formative weeks and months, he or she must be kept from other dogs who are yappy, aggressive, or badly behaved. The dog should also be conditioned to accept being alone in a crate or small room for at least a few hours at a time. Overall it's a lot of hard work, it's easy to mess something up, and it represents a *lot* of time for you to wait before you've got a dog-shaped object that responds to basic commands and that can be taken for walks in public. Is this an amount of time you can afford to invest in a dog before finding out if he or she is Hearing Ear dog potential?

Honeybits passed her CGC at the age of about sixteen months, well short of the eighteen-month mark at which an animal stops behaving like a pup and starts behaving more like an adult dog. By age two, Honeybits's Hearing Ear training was well underway. This happened organically and naturally, and one of the reasons we're so happy is because I was *not* in a hurry to get a fully trained dog. I didn't experience any frustration or impatience, except to the extent that everyone wants the testing to be over and done with. But it still took well over two years of effort to get my service dog.

If you're a professional trainer with appropriate facilities, or if you've got a Hearing Ear dog already in the household and are willing to train one for someone else, there's something to be said for snagging an available pup. You'd be working with a relatively unmarked slate, and you'd know everything about the animal including his or her past experiences. The odds of producing a trained Hearing Ear dog who could pass the Public Access Test would be very high.

If, however, you have *never* had a service animal—or if you've never owned a dog—I wouldn't recommend a puppy unless you're raising him or her with regular input from a trainer. It's important to not turn the puppy into a family pet, or to accidentally reinforce bad habits that make subsequent training difficult. But if you're confident you can raise a puppy, and if you're willing to invest the time bonding and training with the animal, you may just be able to benefit from an extremely strong bond like the one Honeybits and I share.

There's risk associated with raising a puppy, because puppies are not blank slates. They have different levels of energy, intelligence, attentiveness, and disposition to bond with you as a partner. Not every warm, silky ball of fur is going to make a good Hearing Ear dog. The last thing you need to do is to invest two years of time, money, and effort and still not have a dog who can pass the Public Access Test.

If you are looking for a pup who is more likely to be disposed to training, pick the calm, mild-mannered pup who looks at you a lot. If you have a litter of puppies, try snapping your fingers and seeing which ones look at you. Try staring into each pair of sweet, soulful eyes to see which one stares back. Author Alexandra Horowitz identified only one factor that makes one puppy more likely to bond with you and obey you: the disposition to gaze at you. So, if you're looking for a pup to train as a service animal, and you've already selected a breed mix and size that is suitable for a Hearing Ear dog, check out the whole litter. Pick the pup who looks at you and who follows you with his or her eyes. This is the one who secretly wants you as a boss, who thinks you're important, and who will go out of his or her way to please you.

Chapter 8: Gear

This chapter covers some of the equipment you'll need for your service animal. These items are in addition to what you would need for a pet dog.

Leash

Your leash should be thick enough to allow you to control your dog, generally three quarters of an inch across. The leash should be no more than six feet (2 meters) long. It should be flat, and it should be free from ribbons, bows, and adornment. The exception is that you may have "Service Dog" printed down the length of your leash. I prefer a reflective leash since Honeybits and I are often out at night.

You may, if you choose, invest in a "gentle leader" rope that goes around your dog's nose and allows you to deter him or her from sniffing or eating things on the ground or from pulling in a direction you don't want. This is only necessary in the early part of training.

Even if you have a small animal, avoid the decorative half-inch leashes. They do not wear well and they are seldom strong enough to allow you to hoist your dog out of a bad situation or to perform the "emergency pop-up" I describe in the next chapter.

A retractable leash—one that has a handle and a spool of cord or cable—is unacceptable. Nothing says "pet in a vest" quite like a retractable leash. If you're out in public, your dog should be walking at heel or no more than one dog-length ahead of you, with the leash loose.

Harness

A small dog should wear a harness instead of a collar. The harness is vital if you plan to tether your dog into a travel basket, or if you need to lift the dog out of danger. A collar will crush the trachea or windpipe of a dog if the dog's entire weight slams into it suddenly. A fast car stop or even a minor accident can seriously injure or kill a dog who is restrained only by a collar.

Although I like for Honeybits to wear a collar sometimes, I seldom attach a leash to it. The leash is attached to the harness, which she wears *in addition* to a collar, a vest, a poncho, or whatever other clothing is appropriate. Honeybits very rarely pulls at the leash, so her walking behavior is in no way compromised by the use of a harness.

The harnesses I choose for Honeybits tend to have a solid piece across the front and it closes in the back with Velcro, a plastic click lock, and two loops that can be attached to a leash. There is a space for each leg, which means that in the case of an impact the force will be distributed across her shoulders, ribcage, and breastbone depending on the angle. Not one part of the harness is in contact with her neck.

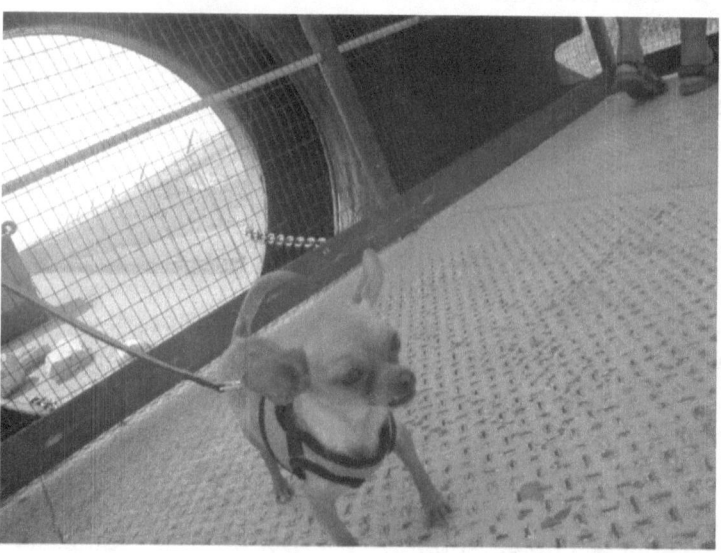

I dislike harnesses that open from the front and that are closed only with Velcro or some kind of decorative attachment. At five pounds, Honeybits is solid muscle and is simply too strong for a front-opening harness. As a puppy, when she weighed only about three and a half pounds and had not yet started obedience training, she consistently burst out of a front-opening harness and went bouncing naked down the block with her little ears flapping. As amusing as it was to the neighborhood children, obviously it didn't work from a safety perspective. Also, it the escape only needed to happen once or twice before her walnut-sized brain went: "Hmm, if I pull and lunge hard enough I can streak the retriever next door *and* make Boss chase me." That could easily have become one of her little puppy goals for every walk, and then part of her usual routine. But I realized that the harness itself was rewarding bad behavior, so I gave it away immediately to a less ambitious dog and went for a rear-closing model. Honeybits lunged for a little bit but gradually realized that she couldn't break free or wiggle out, and accepted that her streaking days were over.

It's important to get a harness that fits your dog. If you choose a smaller dog as your Hearing Ear service animal, make sure the harness you buy is designed for a small dog. This will generally not be a scaled-down version of what larger animals wear, because the straps, clips, and D-rings are out of proportion and so is the thickness of the material. A small dog's harness needs to be strong but lightweight. The one in the above picture is proportioned beautifully, although for hot weather in August in a tropical or subtropical region, I use one consisting of mesh and straps.

Gear Bag

If you're unfortunate enough to be female, you already know how irritating it is to not have pockets built into your clothing and to need somewhere to carry your wallet, your phone, your sunglasses, and everything else you need. You most likely carry a purse already, so when you're out walking your dog you've already noticed that life gets better when you leave the purse behind. Now, double or triple that experience and what you have is a gear bag.

I briefly tried putting everything in my purse, but it didn't work. All that happened was that when I urgently needed something like my keys or a poop bag, I'd have to root, and root, and root through the purse for several seconds before finding what I need. I therefore prefer to have a doggie gear bag.

The best gear bags have a cross-body strap. That allows me to keep both hands free so that I can have one on the dog's leash and the other available to open doors, push a shopping cart, or do other things that require both hands.

Your gear bag should contain everything you need for your dog while you're out. Planning a day outside the house with the dog requires that you spend time thinking about what you're going to need. You don't need to pack up the entire house, but you do need what you plan to use for the day.

Clicker and Treats

If you're in the training phase, you'll need a small "clicker" such as dog trainers use. You can get one at any good pet store, but most professional training companies or dog daycares sell them. They're roughly the size of a key fob and they often come on a wrist loop or cord.

The dog treats can be whatever you wish: little nibbles of something tasty work well if you need to quickly reward something your dog does.

Potty Bags

What you do in your own home is up to you. I've always been disgusted by people who let their animals poop in the yard or in a dog run and who don't clean it up for days. The practice attracts flies and stinks ridiculously. So, I use puppy pads for Honeybits, and don't allow her outside unless she's on a leash. That means I'm present for all the poop. I gather it up in a little plastic bag and toss it into the nearest public garbage can or into the outdoor trash can at my home.

When you're out in public with your dog, it's your duty to clean up the doody. The little bags are inexpensive and they come in rolls. Keep a roll in your car, a roll in your dog gear bag, a roll in your purse, a roll in the house, and a roll everywhere you happen to be.

There are spool-based devices that have a carabiner clip on them. The simplest one is just a pouch with a hole in it where you can pull out one bag at a time. These are fantastic. I use one to clip a roll of poop bags in the car. I've seen other people clip them to purse straps, belts, and gear bags. On a long road trip, the dog sometimes pulls a bag out when she wants to make a pit stop.

Clothing

If your dog will be outside with you in all weather, make sure you protect him or her from the heat or cold. I like to keep a dog sweater or poncho in the car so that if the weather changes suddenly when we're out the Chihuahua can be comfortable. If you carry a gear bag, it's reasonable to keep the clothing in the gear bag.

I prefer to attach Honeybits's winter harness outside of her clothing. If you prefer to use the same kind of harness year-round and to attach it inside clothing, then whatever clothing you pick will have to help communicate that your animal is a service dog. Many people buy vests for their dogs to wear over the harness.

If you want your dog's harness to be under the clothing, thread the leash or the harness attachment points through the hole in the back of the vest. In my opinion, a service dog vest (which generally opens from the front and has no breastbone portion) is not sturdy enough to function as a harness. The vest serves only to identify the animal, not to physically protect him or her.

Tether and Travel Box

A Hearing Ear Dog in particular should learn to ride in a car with a tether. Here's a picture of the system I use with Honeybits.

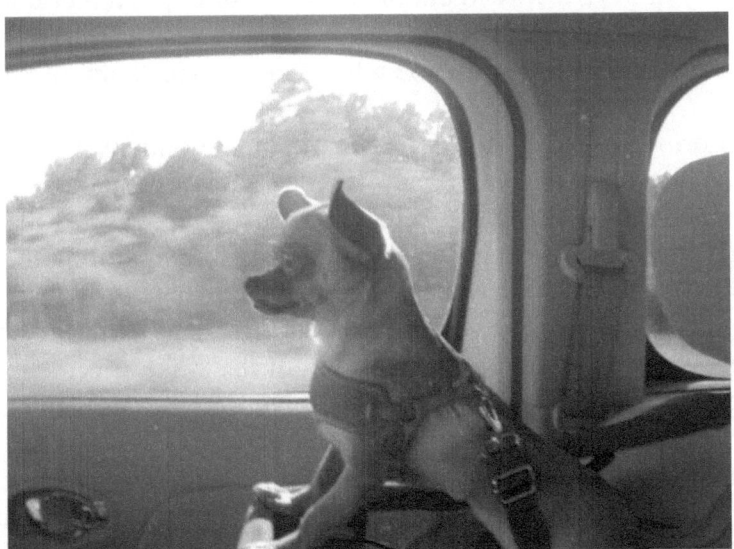

As you can see, she's wearing a travel harness and seated—or in this case standing—in a box strapped to the passenger seat of the car. Her harness is secured to the box itself by means of a strap and a clip. The position of the box is adjustable, and I have it up high enough for her to see out of the car windows and to hear accurately from all directions. Not only does this reduce car sickness, but it allows her to work by pointing to the source of loud noises such as sirens. In a crate in the back seat or the hatch portion of the vehicle, the dog can point all day long but I'm not going to see her.

Here is another scenario in which small dogs are well suited for Hearing Ear work. A large dog cannot safely be kept in the front seat because the weight of the animal will cause the passenger side airbag to enable. This can hurt or even kill a dog, but it is not a risk to Honeybits because her basket is above the level of the seat. The airbag cannot engage. Meanwhile, the box provides some protection and the tether keeps her from being knocked against the side of a rigid kennel or thrown out of the vehicle. Safety-wise, Honeybits's system is a very good compromise that meets the legal requirements for a safety tether in the states that require it. Box assemblies like these, which come complete with an adjustable tether and anchoring straps, are sold by many department stores and pet stores.

Water Escape Tool

Make sure you have a way to cut or release your dog's tether quickly if there's an accident and your car ends up in the water. You'll find it hard to live with yourself if you escape while your service animal drowns.

There's more than one device on the market that contains a cutting blade to release a seatbelt and to smash a window. Buy one and keep it in your car. If you end up in the water, release (or cut) your seatbelt, then release (or cut) your dog's tether. Once everyone is free including the passengers, open the door, bash out a window, or do whatever it takes to make a space out of the car. Shove your dog out first, and let his or her survival skills take over. Then get yourself out of the sinking vehicle. By the time you reach the surface, your dog will have figured out which direction to swim in. Dog-paddle right behind him or her. Then, like the legendary yellow Techichi dogs of Tenochtitlan who guided their Aztec handlers across the river of death into the afterlife, your dog will guide you in the direction of the closest land. Only in this case, you'll both live. Just paddle for your life and follow the dog.

Your water escape tool should be within easy reach of a person in the car. Strap it to your sun visor or find some other place in the car where you can get to it quickly. It should not be buried in your gear bag, your glove box, your purse, or under the seat.

Crate

Most dogs like a den of some kind when they want a quick nap or to hide from the world. A crate is a good way to do this. Many dogs are crate trained, and will sleep in the crate overnight. But you don't want to leave an adult dog in a crate all day long.

I recommend a travel crate for bigger dogs, but a Hearing Ear Dog must be able to see out the window of the car and must be in line of sight of the hearing impaired driver. He or she cannot work in a crate, because one of the things a Hearing Ear Dog should do is to point in the direction of oncoming sirens or other noise. If the dog is in a crate or in the back seat the way most pets travel, you can't see him or her and are not getting the support the dog is trained to provide.

In an airplane, large pet dogs cannot ride in the cabin although pets small enough to fit in carriers are permitted under the seat in front of you. Larger service dogs sit at the feet of the people they serve. A Hearing Ear dog sitting next to your feet in an airplane is not in your direct line of sight and therefore cannot perform pointing work although they are still capable of nudging an ankle or putting a paw on your foot or leg. A Hearing Ear dog tiny enough to be held in your lap is an incredible advantage on a plane, particularly on cross-country or overseas flights of several hours when the flight is delayed and you have to potty the dog on a puppy pad in a miniscule airplane lavatory. However, the dog must remain quiet and with you at all times. The dog cannot roam around the cabin, soil the airplane carpet, or solicit attention from the other passengers. If your dog is a family pet used to soliciting attention from strangers, he or she may require extra training to be calm in an airplane.

Unnecessary Items

You will not need to buy a dog purse, backpack, or carrying system to tote your Hearing Ear Dog around. Service animals walk unless there's a compelling reason for them to be carried. If there's broken glass on the ground or it's a hot summer day and the asphalt is too hot for your dog to walk on, by all means carry your animal. If you're in a cemetery or museum, you may choose to carry the dog not because you're afraid he or she will urinate or defecate inappropriately or damage something, but as proof that he or she did not do so. But you don't have to buy special equipment to do that. If you have that sort of equipment, it actually makes you and your dog look fake.

You won't need a choke collar, a muzzle, or a shock collar. You won't need a pry stick or any kind of discipline tool for negative reinforcement. You won't need a chain, a stake, or an outdoor tethering system because the dog won't be left outdoors for any significant length of time.

Chapter 9: Training Goals

By now you are aware that Hearing Ear dogs, like all service animals, do much more than simply respond to their environment. The training process is not only for the dog: the handler must be able to respond to the dog's cues and to issue the appropriate commands. Dogs are not like cars or motorcycles where if you can operate one you can pretty much figure out all of them. Ideally the dog and the handler will work together from the very beginning. This chapter discusses what the training is like and which behaviors a Hearing Ear dog needs to display.

Once you have a dog who is young, healthy, housebroken, and through the screening process, you can begin the training process. This chapter will introduce the various training goals and benchmarks that apply to service dog training in general and to Hearing Ear dog training in particular.

Obedience

All dogs, even pets, should be taught basic obedience as puppies. They should learn to sit, lie down, stay, wait as a handler walks through a door, and walk on a loose leash, stopping when you stop and turning when you turn. They should sit or lie down still for petting and examination, they should be able to maintain a neutral attitude and pass a new person or a dog without pulling, lunging, barking, or fleeing. They should be able to hold a sit and stay. A service dog should be able to do all these things, and more.

Your service dog should drop or avoid a forbidden item, such as a morsel of food on the ground, if you give the command. You should also have an "out" command that will cause the dog to drop whatever is in his or her mouth, even if it's food. Honeybits is so well disciplined that I can reach into her mouth and pull out a piece of food without worrying about being bitten. For a ball or other large "play" item, I have a command that will make her release it.

There are two kinds of recall training your dog should be able to perform. He or she should be able to maintain a sit or down position while you walk to a distance and then come to you when summoned. The dog should also respond to an attention-getting command that causes him or her to stop what he or she is doing and come to you immediately. These might be line of sight commands, audible commands such as a leg slap, whistle, or finger snap, or some combination of both. My recall signal is a variation of the American Sign Language word for "dog".

Eating and Drinking

A well trained service animal will not take food from any person besides you, unless you give the word. If there's something edible on the ground and you tell the dog to leave it, he or she will not gobble the morsel up. This prevents your dog from accidentally (or deliberately) being poisoned or from eating something wormy or unwholesome that makes him or her sick.

Some service animals are trained to eat only on command, when presented with food and commanded by the handler to eat. This level of training obviously requires that the dog not be food-aggressive or the kind of animal who bolts down everything in sight.

Potty Training

If you can teach the dog to urinate or defecate on command it's an incredibly useful skill to have because you can "empty" the dog before going into a building. Larger dogs do tend to have more deliberate control over their bowels and bladders. Some animals, if praised and rewarded for eliminating in response to a command word, try their best when you issue the command word simply because they want the treat.

I've trained Honeybits to make use of puppy pads. As I mentioned earlier, I can easily carry a puppy pad with me to put on the floor of a restroom stall or an airplane toilet so that the dog and I can do our business at the same time. I flush any solids, and the puppy pad absorbs urine. This is a very good strategy for a small dog, particularly on an airplane.

Whatever solution you select, you must develop a way to empty the dog before you go into a cemetery, a house of worship, an airport, or any other place where you can't readily duck out for a quick potty break. Your dog can't tell the difference between a cemetery and a city park, and you must be the one in control of whether your dog squats there. This is especially true if you go to dog beaches or other dog-friendly places where there's a designated relief area.

Specialized Crowd Techniques for Small Dogs

Taking a small dog out in a crowd can be a challenge but I've developed four specialized techniques that I believe will help. The general idea is that to create safe space *for* your dog, all you need to do is to create well defended space *above* your dog. I practice and train all these techniques with Honeybits.

If you carry a bag of some sort for all your dog related documentation and gear, don't make it a backpack. Make it a cross-body sling bag, because that extends the width of your body and provides a dog's width and dog's length worth of overhead protection. A person who bumps sideways into you will hit your bag, but his or her feet won't be anywhere near your dog.

The Modified Heel

When you're in a crowded space with a small dog, you must modify the heel technique so that nobody steps on your dog. In heavy foot traffic, where people have strollers, wheelchairs, and rapid changes of direction and speed, it's simply not safe to have your animal beside or behind you. If he or she will be providing alert services, the dog must be in your line of sight. It is therefore appropriate for the dog to be about a step ahead of you, to one side. This should never turn into a situation where your dog pulls ahead past the end of the aisle in a grocery store, because you need to be able to physically protect your dog in a crowd.

This modified "fuss" (the German term means "foot") is not the heeling technique taught in obedience, rally, Schutzhund, or agility. In those sports, the dog is expected to follow to the side of the handler and slightly beside. He or she is often in physical contact with the handler's leg. For crowd purposes with a small dog, that's a very bad place to be. If you stop or turn suddenly, you could easily step on a small dog. Also, whereas a large dog is in contact with your knee or thigh, a small dog is in contact with your ankle. Ankles don't move smoothly through space.

They stay planted, then lift as you take each step. For this reason, it's dangerous for a little dog to be in a conventional "fuss" position. A heel in which your dog leads slightly on the leash side, by no more than a dog length so that your entire dog is within your line of sight, is safer in my opinion than the conventional fuss. You can keep your eyes on your dog and ensure he or she can move without stepping into danger.

The Elbow

In a crowd, your primary goal will be to prevent your dog from being stepped on by other people. Being stepped on is a risk for tiny dogs, and it's a reason they learn not to get underfoot in the kitchen or around the house where you might turn or back up unexpectedly. In a crowd, your dog must watch out for you *and* for others. So, take advantage of the fact that you occupy space, and use your body to create an umbrella-like space under which your service dog may shelter.

Human beings tend to be widest at the shoulders or hips, not at their feet. They seldom stand with their feet shoulder width apart, and they almost never walk that way. Therefore, at knee to foot level there's generally a good hand's span of lateral distance between the vertical line down from the shoulder or hip and the point at which a human's foot touches the floor.

Moving forward or backward, people instinctively keep their feet within a couple inches of their center mass, and the great news is that center mass is right in the torso. (The things a person learns after decades of martial arts...) Therefore, to keep people's feet away from your dog it is generally sufficient to keep their torso away from the space immediately above your dog. This makes it physically impossible for people to step on the dog by accident.

When in a line or crowd where someone may back up suddenly, I take my leash hand, fold it in toward my breastbone, and stick my elbow out forward, rolling my shoulder forward as I do so. This gives me about sixteen inches, and if I lean slightly toward the people who may step backward, they will bump into a sharp elbow before their feet get anywhere near my dog. This also pulls the leash back toward my chest, shortening the length Honeybits has to work with and informing her that she needs to be close to me.

The Step-In

From time to time, your dog will be at risk from a threat on the ground. This might be a runaway shopping cart, a large and hostile dog, or any number of things. Your small dog will probably instinctively try to either protect you or to run behind you. With Honeybits I established myself early as her protector, so she tends to either tuck in behind me or freeze in place as I step between her and the threat.

One of your feet and legs will be closer to the threat than the other. This is the leg I will call the "blocking" leg. To perform a step-in, first take your weight off your blocking leg. Pull on the leash in the direction opposite to the threat, which is where you are shifting your weight. Then put the blocking leg between your dog and the threat, step down, and pretend you're a wall. Make eye contact with the threat if necessary.

The Emergency Pop-Up

For emergencies I have perfected what I call an "emergency pop-up". It's exactly what it sounds like: a sudden vertical yank that causes the harness-wearing dog to fly up into the air to about shoulder level, where I can snag her with one hand and pull her close to me. Honeybits, when popped up, has been trained to turn toward me and scramble toward my shoulder. This makes it easier to hold her with one arm while I use my feet and my other hand to do whatever else needs to be done.

The emergency pop-up is something a large, aggressive animal often doesn't expect, because the small dog suddenly moves in a very unusual direction. It's also fast, and it can be executed without changing your foot position. You can use it in conjunction with the step-in but it is extremely effective on its own. It's allowed me to snatch Honeybits out of the way of a suddenly-reversing truck in the French Quarter of New Orleans, where we came within inches of being crushed.

Disability Specific Training

One of the requirements for a dog to be a service dog is that he or she must assist you with tasks related to your disability. Hearing Ear dogs alert their handlers to things in their environment they need to be aware of. This might include people trying to get your attention, loud noises, people at the door, a crying baby, or a ringing phone. It might include a pointing behavior, nudging or tapping you to get your attention, or simply entering your line of sight. Your dog may have to wake you up out of a sound sleep or selectively disobey you to get your attention and warn you of a hazard.

Most trainers teach the dog at least four separate alert or disability compensation behaviors. Honeybits helps me drive by pointing at loud noises, and she's trained to wake me up if she hears a fire alarm.

The dog must generalize the alert behavior and understand that he or she must apply it in a variety of situations, some of which aren't covered in the training. Here's an example of a generalized behavior. In December of 2019, before she had passed the Public Access Test and in the middle of her training, Honeybits saved the house from burning down. There was a fire in the kitchen I was unaware of because something had spilled in the oven. The tiny Chihuahua came sprinting into the office area of my house, where I was at work on the computer, and tapped me insistently with her paw. When she had my attention, she ran in the direction of the kitchen, paused to make sure I was getting up and following, and led me right to the problem. The fire was small enough for me to be able to put it out. Another minute, and it probably wouldn't have been.

Training Customized for the Handler's Lifestyle

There are people who lose their jobs due to hearing loss, but I'm lucky: I can still work, even with my disability, because I'm in a line of work where I can get by with lip reading, occasional amplification, and communication mostly in writing. I can still drive and participate in the work world, and I hope to continue working for many years to come. Since I mostly live alone (my daughter grew up and moved out), I can't rely on human beings to let me know if something important is happening that I can't hear. I can also enjoy outdoor life. I'm a fiend for national parks, I take a lot of road trips, and I travel for work. The services that Honeybits provides allow me to enjoy a very full and active life.

In the early fall of 2018, I took an epic road trip with Honeybits. Over two and a half weeks, we crisscrossed New Mexico, Texas, Oklahoma, Arkansas, Tennessee, Mississippi, Alabama, and Louisiana. Sometimes we camped, and sometimes we stayed in dog-friendly hotels or in a timeshare. I wasn't afraid to drive thousands of miles solo or to camp alone in a deserted recreation facility, because Honeybits kept me safe. She gave me the exact information I needed to make decisions, drive safely, and step out of the way of a suddenly-reversing truck in the French Quarter of New Orleans. In the summer of 2019, I took the dog on a Rocky Mountain trip through Utah, Idaho, Montana, North and South

Dakota, Wyoming, and Colorado. We went canoeing on a quiet, flat part of the Colorado River near Moab, Utah.

Because I travel a lot, I need support so that I don't sleep through another hotel fire alarm. (The first two were more than enough.) I can buy all kinds of adaptive products for the home, including doorbells, alarm clocks, phones, and smoke detectors designed for hearing-impaired people. A few hotels have strobes attached to their smoke detectors, but I have yet to see a hotel room with a flashing doorbell or a vibrating alarm clock. I can bring my own alarm clock when I travel, however when I'm camping in a tent there's nowhere to plug it in. Accordingly, Honeybits has been trained to alert me to the same things as all the audible alarms and ringtones that fill up a hearing person's world.

Depending on your lifestyle, you may not need a silent alert or assistance in a car. If you don't travel, or if you travel only with other people, you may be able to get by with *them* performing the alert functions that Honeybits provides for me. But if you ever have to function alone, then a very simple thing such as ordering pizza can become difficult without electronic aid or four-footed help. When I place an order for pizza, Honeybits points at the phone when it rings with the restaurant's confirmation call. I'm not physically capable of hearing a knock at the door even with my hearing aids turned all the way up, so Honeybits tells me when the delivery driver arrives. She can do this for me no matter where we are, including in a hotel room.

The very minimum I would suggest, when training your Hearing Ear dog, is to train in door alerts, a special fire alarm alert that involves waking you up when you're asleep, an alert for the alarm clock, and an alert for an oncoming siren. Honeybits also has ways of telling me when there's someone behind me, when food on the stove is boiling over, exactly *who* is at the door, and whether there's someone approaching my tent.

If you live with family members or other people, it may be useful to train your dog to go for help if you're having a medical emergency. I myself didn't seek out this form of training for Honeybits because I live alone. Because her training was customized for me and for my particular needs, we didn't have to invest time and effort in a behavior that cannot be effectively practiced and that will most likely never be used.

A dog who wakes you up for a fire alarm could easily save your life. A dog who wakes you up when you miss the alarm clock can save your job. A dog who relieves your spouse of alerting and caregiving duties, so that the love of your life no longer feels like a babysitter, can save your marriage. A dog who informs you of a kitchen fire can save the house from burning down.

Justification for Formal Training

Much of a Hearing Ear Dog's work is in the home. While visiting Memphis, Tennessee, I met a Deaf woman who had dogs of her own, but who had never considered training any of them to perform Hearing Ear work. The dogs understood sign language and were very obedient, yet because my new acquaintance traveled with a family member who did the driving and the answering of doors and telephones, my new acquaintance was already getting the assistance she needed. For her, it was easier to arrange for one family member to take care of her dogs while she was on vacation and for another to accompany her. You could say that she didn't need a Hearing Ear dog because she already had a Hearing Ear human. Yet not everybody has such an effective human support system, and *not everyone likes having people around while traveling.*

Plenty of people who are born and raised Deaf have access to interpreters, but do you really want to cover room, board, and payment for a pair of interpreters to accompany you on multi-day trips? For engagements longer than two hours, a team of interpreters really are necessary because it's physically exhausting to keep up with people who talk quickly. An interpreter, when traveling, can also perform most of the functions of a Hearing Ear dog. But, even if you can afford to support a team of interpreters or have a third party that helps you to pay, do you really want to share your hotel room, recreational vehicle, or tent with a relative stranger?

A dog obviously can't sign or fingerspell to you, but they do provide mobile alert services.

One of the most depressing things about life with a disability—any disability—is that travel becomes an order of magnitude more difficult and potentially dangerous. No law requires us to limit ourselves to our homes and places of work, but ask yourself these questions:

What if driving were no longer dangerous or frightening?

What if it was safe to sleep in a different city by yourself?

What if you could go camping without relying on somebody else to take care of you?

What if you could be part of a road trip group without worrying about being a burden to others?

What if you didn't have to pay extra for someone to accompany you on a trip? You could afford to travel twice as much.

What if you didn't have to stay in a bad marriage, or live with a resentful or even abusive relative, or compromise your style of living simply because you "need" other people around to compensate for your disability?

What if people came up to you and started positive conversations without trying to sell you something, simply because they notice and like you, and think you are friendly?

What if you didn't have to be isolated anymore?

You can have all of these things. You can hold onto the freedom and independence you've got just a little while longer, OR you can reach out and take more independence than you ever thought possible.

Training for Multiple Disabilities

If you have more than one disability for which a service dog would be useful, it is wise to select a dog with attributes necessary for all the tasks. A person with both PTSD and hearing loss, for example, needs a dog large enough to perform PTSD related tasks.

A service dog who has already been trained for another task can easily be cross-trained as a Hearing Ear dog without compromising his or her existing service dog skills. I use the word "easily" because much of the training work that goes into a service dog involves obedience and the behaviors necessary to function in public and to pass the Public Access Test. That effort obviously does not need to be repeated.

Compared to other kinds of service dog training, alert training is some of the easiest, fastest, and least expensive to perform. Trainers use reward based techniques such as "capturing" and "shaping" to capitalize on a dog's natural responses to changes in his or her environment. The clicker-based training discussed by Karen Pryor in *Don't Shoot the Dog—The New Art of Teaching and Training* relies on what psychologists call "operant conditioning". An animal who associates approval and reward with a click will deliberately repeat the behavior that produced the click and the reward. This is a humane and fun way of training, and because it contains only positive reinforcement many dogs consider it to be a type of play. A dog who is used to learning new behaviors can sometimes absorb a new technique in just one day, however weeks of repetition are necessary to "reinforce" the behavior so that the dog remembers it in the long term.

A Bigger Bang for the Buck

Because alert behaviors are the easiest to capture and shape through operant conditioning, training a dog for alert functions is far faster and easier than training one for, say, the intensive guide work done by a seeing-eye dog. Indeed, a healthy young dog who has already earned the Canine Good Citizen title can often get through the rest of the training in six months of training, with one to two hours a week of attention from a professional trainer and the remainder of the effort coming from the handler.

A Hearing Ear Dog need not be bred deliberately and trained from puppyhood. An owner-surrendered dog or an animal from a foster-based rescue can be just as effective, if they have the suitable temperament and circumstances. They are available for far less than a purebred puppy would cost. In a for-profit training organization, anything that reduces the net price to the customer is something that makes sense to consider. In the not-for-profit domain, success isn't measured in terms of profit but in terms of the number of people served with the available budget. Anything that improves the turnaround time by allowing a beneficiary to receive a dog earlier or more cheaply is a good idea *provided it doesn't result in a poorly trained or badly behaved service animal, and provided the beneficiary or customer isn't misled into investing time and money into a dog who will not be capable of performing the appropriate service work.*

Chapter 10: Training Techniques

Modern trainers use reward-based "positive reinforcement" training. This is not solely out of consideration for the dog or a desire to be kind and humane—although each of those motivations is worthy in its own right—so much as out of practicality. Positive reinforcement training works much more quickly and more reliably than the old-fashioned methods. Anyone who is in the business of producing functional service animals (either for profit or otherwise) needs to do the job as quickly and cheaply as possible, without sacrificing quality. Positive reinforcement training causes the animal to learn behaviors and change behaviors quickly and permanently, and to develop a desire to perform the behaviors whenever the opportunity arises. You see, it turns out that animals are a little bit like people: the best way to get them to do something is to make them *want* to do it.

The Case for Positive Reinforcement

The word "reinforcement" comes from B. F. Skinner, an early psychologist who noticed that people and animals tend to mentally associate things that occur at the same time and in the same place. Human beings, for example, often remember the fragrance worn by a romantic partner. If they catch a whiff of that fragrance, they will be reminded of that partner even if he or she is not present. Likewise, the smell of a well-cooked holiday feast or the sight of a delicious meal makes people feel hungry. Advertisers take advantage of these mental associations to sell goods and services.

People and animals also respond to incentives. They might be positive incentives, such as rewards, or they might be negative incentives, such as punishments. If you reward a person or animal for a specific behavior, the odds are very high that he or she will repeat it in hope of getting the reward. Rewarding a desired behavior on the spot, which is known as "capturing", is great for taking advantage of a natural or instinctive behavior. But for the more complex behaviors necessary for service work, a behavior must be "shaped".

Skinner recognized that the kind of feedback presented to a person or animal during training could "reinforce" a behavior. The idea behind rewarding good behavior, for example, is that people or animals tend to do more of the things we reward and fewer of the things we punish... *if*, of course, they associate the reward or punishment with the specific action we want them to associate it with. To make that association work, it's vital that the reinforcement occur immediately after the key decision you want to reinforce. The longer you wait before providing a reward or punishment, the less likely an animal (or human) is to associate it with the action you're trying to reinforce.

Why Punishment Produces Unreliable Results

Punishment doesn't produce uniform or unreliable results even within a species that responds to it in general. If it did, humanity would have figured out an effective law enforcement strategy by now. There are always some individuals—and in certain species, *most* individuals—who simply don't associate a punishment with the specific thing you're punishing them for. Even if you catch them in the act and punish them immediately, the message you want them to get ("stop doing that and never do it again") is not the message they internalize.

I'm going to use human behavior as an example. Suppose two teenaged girls are in the high school principal's office. Both of whom are getting detention because they wore something that violated the school dress code. (I'm using girls in this case instead of boys for two reasons. First, nearly all dress code restrictions are directed against female students as opposed to male students. Second, most clothing marketed to young women is flimsy and revealing enough to violate at least one school dress code, whereas young men have to work exceptionally hard to find such a garment.) Suppose the two girls broke the same rule, in the same way, on the same day. Both are aware that their offense is trivial in the grand scheme of things—nobody died or went to the hospital—and both are aware that the punishment they're receiving is grossly out of proportion with the damage or risk created by the broken rule. They have always known about the rule, but they have both seen other students get away with breaking it, and they are aware that it does not apply to male students. Indeed, they have gotten away with breaking the rule once or twice. But today the rule is being enforced.

Girl #1 understands that the rule existed long before she came around, that she knew about the rule, and that she knew she was breaking it. She is aware that the rule isn't always enforced and that some students are exempt from it due to factors beyond her control. But she interprets her punishment as a direct result of what *she* did. She learns from the experience and adapts her behavior to ensure she follows the dress code and never gets in trouble again. It's not necessarily that she believes that everything that happens to her is somehow her fault—she is fully capable of explaining how her decisions were influenced by others. She might point to the dress code itself, which is perhaps inherently unfair and sexist because it focuses almost exclusively on restricting female attire instead of male attire. She might point out that the dress code is difficult to follow with the clothing actually available in her price range. She might take note of teachers or staff members who come to the school dressed in ways that violate the dress code, and she may point at the lax enforcement of the code in the recent past. These things, which do not necessarily justify her decision, created an environment in which she felt as though violating the dress code was a reasonable idea. She is still able to draw a distinction between the factors in her environment and the particular decision she made to flout the rules, because she recognizes it as a decision. She adjusts her behavior and never again violates the dress code.

Girl #2 understands that the rule existed on paper, but that it was never actually enforced, so for all intents and purposes it didn't exist unless an authority figure *wanted* to enforce it. Every time she saw someone get away with breaking it, she interpreted it as further evidence that the rule wasn't real. The fact that she is being singled out and punished while other people continue to get away with breaking the rule is, to her, further evidence that the rule itself is arbitrary. She's being punished, but the rule is not the reason why. In her mind, the teacher has simply decided to punish her, and her mind fills in another reason. Maybe she decides the teacher dislikes her, or maybe there's another reason to blame someone else for the consequences of her decision to break the rule. She never accepts the dress code as legitimate and retaliates by flouting authority in other ways. She just learns how to do what she wants without getting caught. This strategy may work in the artificial school world of arbitrary punishments, but if she develops the habit of pushing the limits, flouting authority, and ignoring rules she doesn't wish to follow, she may have difficulty functioning in the adult world where there are bad consequences to pushing other people's boundaries, ignoring tax and traffic laws, and failing to respect in-laws, employers, and police officers.

Even within our own species, if we deal out the same punishment to two different individuals, we frequently don't get the reform we're looking for and the end result is extremely unpredictable. If a human being doesn't reliably draw the conclusion we're looking for—"I am being punished because I did *this*", an animal is even less likely to do so. Punishment, especially when it's after the fact, is often something the animal associates with *you* rather than with whatever behavior you're trying to correct. They may simply learn to do the forbidden behavior only when you're not around.

Most wild animals think more like Girl #2 than like Girl #1. Most humans, and many dogs, think more like Girl #1 especially if they have been trained and socialized a lot. But just as with human beings, dogs have a range of dispositions, and sometimes the behavior you think you're punishing isn't the one the dog associates with the punishment.

Swatting a puppy with a rolled-up newspaper for peeing on the carpet is just as stupid as it is cruel. From the dog's perspective, it looks like this: "I have been just minding my own business for a long time: I ate, I drank some water, I found a comfortable place to pee, but Boss has come home and she's angry. She rubbed my nose in my pee and she hit me. I'm going to have to avoid her in the future, and maybe find a better place to empty my bladder. Her closet might be better: there are lots of smelly shoes in there and some funny-looking ones she calls 'Manolos'. I'll pee on those next."

A luckier dog whose handler follows a positive reinforcement process has an experience like this: "Boss has come home, she saw the pee spot, and she's cleaning it up. There's no pee odor left so obviously this isn't a good place to empty my bladder. But, you know what is? That nice puppy pad she's set up for me. Last time I peed on one like it, she gave me a treat and called me a good boy. Maybe if I pee there, I can make that happen again."

Consider what happens when a puppy gets hold of a nice, crunchy pen with a full ink cartridge. It's the perfect size to chew. It's crunchy on the outside and liquid on the inside. Also, it gets a reaction out of the dog handler. But, what happens next?

A punitive dog handler will become angry, demand that the dog come over and give up the new toy. But would *you* approach an obviously angry boss who demands that you give up the good thing you've found? Or would you slow down if your angry boss decided to chase you? Most likely you'd flee. If you were a dog, you might enjoy a game of Chase the Puppy in which you lead Boss on a merry chase through the living room, chomping as you go. You incidentally learn that if you want to initiate a chase game in the future, all you have to do is to grab a forbidden item, taunt your boss with it, and then take off. If the game gets too serious and Boss gets too angry, you might flee in earnest and it may not occur to you to drop what you're carrying.

A handler who uses positive reinforcement will not let the dog bait him or her into a game of Chase the Puppy, no matter how fragile or valuable the hostage item might be. Instead, the handler brings out a treat or a favorite toy and proposes a trade. The dog willingly gives up the hostage item in a better condition than it would have been after an extended chase and scuffle. He or she might learn that approaching with a key item may prompt you to offer a higher-value treat in exchange. The dog might even initiate a game or training session where you work some "out" or "drop it" exercises. But approaching you never feels unsafe because you don't act like you're crazy, out of control, or highly aroused.

Some dogs who are taught to "trade" forbidden items for treats or higher-value toys may go out of their way to find or collect things you've swapped for treats in the past. They may bring you what they think will be good barter items. This is kind of cute, and it's far better than trying to chase a small, slippery dog.

A dog raised with positive reinforcement techniques bonds better with his or her handler and lives in a secure, high-trust environment. He or she associates the handler with attention, affection, play, and treats.

Natural Consequences as an Alternative to Punishment

The best way to correct an undesirable behavior in a human *or* an animal is to ensure that the subject learns that *the behavior won't get them what they want, no matter when or how they do it*. This, incidentally, is how puppies are socialized by their mothers and pack mates. If someone nips too hard, the nipped party yelps and the game is over. The game does not continue. Likewise, if Honeybits gets too excited around guests, I put her into my bedroom to settle down for a while.

In the animal world, if you play too roughly with a playmate the game stops immediately. If you bite instead of nursing, you don't get to continue your meal. If you behave rudely toward other animals, they don't want to be around you and have ways to make their objections known. If for some reason you're not wanted in the pack, you have the option of going it alone or joining another pack. The rest of the pack learns to get by without you. Only in the human world are individuals forced to continue to interact with those who actively harm them or who prey upon them. Disapproval from the rest of the pack and the disappearance of the thing you want seldom works with human adults, but it is a very effective way to get puppies to conform.

Humanity has all kinds of disordered behavior that comes in part from having a set of people whose bad behavior is tolerated or even encouraged while everyone else is artificially prevented from either escaping or administering enough correction to make the bad behavior stop. We have addictions, for example, along with the entitlement-minded nonsense that the media has dubbed "affluenza". We have adults in their thirties and forties who, despite being able-bodied and of sound mind, refuse to work for an income and are supported by their elderly parents. There are entire books devoted to different kinds of enabling behavior that begin as well-intentioned attempts to help a human who is self-destructing, but that end up perpetuating the problem. As a species, we aren't good at enforcing group standards. But dogs are. A mother dog generally manages to raise pups that don't bite and that are mannerly toward other dogs.

Environmental Control as an Alternative to Punishment

In *How to Raise the Perfect Dog*, Cesar Millan introduces a very good idea about how to raise a puppy by using positive reinforcement. His key insight in the book is that it's easier to shape an animal's behavior by creating an environment in which the puppy isn't punished for "wrong" choices because the opportunity to make wrong choices doesn't exist while opportunities to make "right" choices (and to be rewarded for them) are plentiful. Millan suggests that, instead of letting the puppy or dog roam free and do whatever comes to mind, it's better to control the animal's environment and keep things simple at first until the desired habits are established. Then the dog's territory can gradually be expanded. I used this strategy with Honeybits and was rewarded with a Chihuahua—said to be one of the most difficult dogs to train—who can be allowed the run of the house while I'm at work. The strategies proposed in *How to Raise the Perfect Dog* emphasize controlling the dog's environment and providing lots of positive examples and positive reinforcement. It did not emphasize punitive or dominance-enforcement techniques.

Consider, for example, the process of potty training. If a puppy is kept in a relatively small pen but is taught to urinate in a specific place and rewarded for doing so, the puppy will continue to urinate in that place even if the pen suddenly becomes larger, provided the rewards are continued for the desired behavior but withheld if the puppy urinates anywhere but in the desired place. The pup will do what produces the reward until the behavior becomes habitual, at which point the rewards are gradually phased out. The puppy cannot urinate on the bedroom carpet because he or she is not given the opportunity to *be* on the carpet until the habit of peeing in the designated place is fully formed and consistent even without the reward. Millan describes a process of gradually expanding a puppy's territory to include a larger pen, a room, an outdoor kennel, and then eventually the rest of the house. By the time the pup encounters a rug or the carpeted living room, it will not occur to him or her to make a mess there.

For an environmental control strategy to work, you must provide the animal with a living situation that is stable, predictable, and fairly simple especially at first. The complexity should increase gradually as the animal matures and develops the behaviors you want while reducing or eliminating the behaviors you don't want. This process is identical to the way dogs and wolves raise their young in a pack scenario, and the way parents tend to raise their children. Regular mealtimes, consistency in terms of a regular caregiver, routines, playmates, and expectations are just as beneficial to animals as they are to children. In a stable environment, it becomes far easier for an animal or child to predict what a peer, authority figure, or family member will do in response to his or her action. When the environment becomes too chaotic and unpredictable—and the threshold varies from one person to the next—both animals and human beings go into a survival mode wherein they are incapable of doing anything but reacting to whatever crisis is occurring at the moment. They develop maladaptive behaviors to help them avoid what hurts or frightens them. These behaviors often become habitual and make it difficult for the animal or human to function in a more normal environment.

The environmental control strategy is useful because it isolates cause and effect. Without a good idea about what is "normal", it's hard to determine just what changes you made that caused a difference in your environment, or whether the thing that changed was related to you at all. Service dog training continues well beyond where a normal pet owner would stop, simply because a service dog must stay mellow and controlled in a variety of chaotic and unpredictable environments.

Dogs have to be taught that the undesirable behavior won't get them what they want, that they can't get what they want by waiting until you're out of the room to do it, and that they *can* get what they want by doing something different. They also have to learn that there are predictable bad things that happen—things, by the way, that have nothing to do with whether you're nearby or involved—when they do something they shouldn't. Sometimes you have to make it easy to be a "good" cat, dog, or bird by controlling the animal's environment so that their behavior options are limited until the habits you consider desirable are well established.

Positive Reinforcement Techniques

There are five major components to positive reinforcement training: rewarding, luring, marking, capturing, and shaping.

Rewarding

"Rewarding" is the process of giving your dog something that motivates him or her. Most dogs like small, edible treats but some are toy-oriented and prefer a quick game of tug-of-war or fetch. If you have a strong bond with your dog, you yourself are the reward: the dog wants your attention, your gaze, your kind word, and maybe some praise and petting. I find much of the progress I've made with Honeybits has come out of our bond. She genuinely wants to interact with me and communicate with me.

To any dog, certain treats or rewards have a higher value than others. If you are fortunate enough to have a Chihuahua, *you* are the greatest reward. Snuggles or praise from you are often more motivating than food. To most large working dogs, food is more interesting than toys. But even within the food category, individual animals have their favorites. Learn what your dog's preferred reward is, and have both high-value and low-value treats on hand.

Over the course of training, rewards are gradually phased out but they never become entirely obsolete. One of the interesting things Skinner noticed about his pigeons and rats is that they, like humans, repeat behaviors for longer if the reward is occasional or intermittent. If a behavior is rewarded one day but the rewards stop completely the next day and do not resume, the animal will often abandon the trained behavior.

Luring

"Luring" is a means of using a reward to get the animal to come or to move about. Dogs are nose-driven creatures. They will often follow a smelly treat into a crate, or a car, or another new environment. When they enjoy the treat, or even a meal, in their new environment without anything startling or unpleasant happening, animals gradually become accustomed to their new surroundings. This is a technique often used in crate-training, place-training, and specialized disability assistance tasks that require an animal to assume an unusual position.

For a young puppy, sitting on command is not a natural behavior, so trainers often use a treat to lure or trick the puppy into sitting. Luring is a technique the trainer uses to stimulate an animal's interest in the place, object, or position. It should not be used to train in a complex task, because there's a risk that the dog will never learn the task and will only begin or complete the behavior if there's a lure involved.

Marking

"Marking" is the process of identifying the specific thing an animal is doing, and calling his or her attention to it, *at the time the animal does that thing*. There are positive markers that identify the behavior as good (and worthy of a reward), and there are negative markers that identify the behavior as bad (and not approved of by the trainer). A negative marker is not a punishment but an identification of a behavior as undesirable.

A positive marker can be any kind of word, signal, or sound. A sound or word of some kind is desirable because the dog will notice it even if he or she is looking away. Most professional trainers use a "clicker": a small device that is said to produce an audible click that is not similar to any of the sounds human beings use when speaking. I find that when I push the button on a clicker, it releases something inside the mechanism that generates the kind of vibration I associate with snapping plastic. Other people have assured me that the click is audible, and the dog will definitely look at the clicker especially once he or she has associated it with a reward. The timing of the click is definitely precise. Whereas it might take us a second or so to get a word out, and if we're talking with someone else we may not wish to speak, a click is discreet and unique. It means "I approve of what you're doing".

At the beginning a dog's training, the trainer or handler will "load" the clicker by using operant conditioning straight out of B. F. Skinner's playbook. He or she will offer the animal a high value treat while clicking the clicker. Then the handler will click and immediately offer a reward. In this way, the dog learns that the clicker means something good: a treat is imminent. Gradually, the handler can separate the treat and the reward by a period of a few seconds. The animal then starts to notice that the treat comes after the click. He or she starts to become interested in actions that might produce a click. From that point onward, the click gets the dog's attention even at a short distance. This is an example of a positive marker.

A negative marker is similar to the warning sound made by a mother dog to correct a wayward pup. It is a noise that means "I do not approve of what you are doing". If you say "uh-uh" to a puppy, that puppy will momentarily pause in what he or she is doing, and do something else for at least a second. If you're smart and prepared, you take advantage of the pause to remove the temptation and show the puppy what you *do* want, perhaps by luring or by giving an alternate command. This will redirect the animal's attention and behavior to something you like better.

Shaping

Anyone who has played "hot and cold" with a child understands shaping. In the "hot and cold" game, one player identifies an object in the room, possibly a hidden object, and the other player has to guess which object it is. The guesser walks around the room and the first player calls out "hot" or "cold" depending on whether the guesser is moving toward the object, or away from it. The word "hot" is a positive marker, and the word "cold" is a negative marker.

To use shaping with a dog, first reward a natural behavior that approximates what you want. If you want the dog to climb into a box, first use click-and-reward techniques when the dog looks at the box. After a few repetitions, reward the dog for moving toward the box, touching the box, and eventually looking inside or putting a paw inside.

Eventually, to get more clicks and treats, your dog will get into the box of his or her own volition.

You can also use shaping to build up a desired command response, gradually refining the dog's behavior by rewarding specific details and by withholding the click or reward otherwise. A clever, well-motivated dog who knows to associate the marking click with a treat responds to a marking click with: "what did I just do? I will do more of that."

Attention-Getting Correction

Sometimes your dog does something you don't want him or her to do. He or she could be following an interesting scent, or doing something instinctive but impolite by human standards. Normal dog behaviors such as burrowing into the freshly washed laundry or trying to steal pizza off the coffee table don't go over well in a human household. So, in addition to marking things you approve of, you must have a way to convey your disapproval of whatever thing your dog is doing *at the precise moment he or she is doing it*. You must also have a way to get your dog's attention when he or she is absorbed with something else in his or her environment that is more interesting than paying attention to you. There are three kinds of attention-getting corrections: negative markers, attention recalls, and physical redirection. If the conditions are right, you can also allow the dog to experience the natural consequences of bad behavior, provided you do not endanger the dog, or yourself, in the process.

Negative Markers

A negative marker is a signal, generally an audible signal, that means "I do not approve of what you are doing". It is not, in itself, a punishment. It is simply the first warning before consequences occur. A mother dog uses a sound similar to an "uh-uh" when a puppy is misbehaving. Puppies instinctively respond to an "uh-uh" kind of sound by stopping whatever they are doing at the moment. "Uh-uh", as a dog-loving friend of mine once told me, is a word in Dog language much like "Hsssst" is a word in Cat. If you use a verbal marker that resembles what the puppy is instinctively disposed to recognize as something that comes from an authority figure, you can take advantage of the puppy's pause to redirect the puppy's attention.

In the dog world, ignoring the first word of warning has consequences. A puppy who plays too roughly and who ignores the mother's "uh-uh" or a playmate's yip of pain will find itself removed from the game if he or she persists. Ignoring the signals from other dogs, some of which are nonverbal, can often cause the encounter to escalate. For this reason, it's important to socialize your dog with other dogs well enough to ensure that he or she does not stare, walk directly up to a frightened or tail-tucked dog, or continue to get into another dog's space.

A mother dog or wolf provides escalating correction. Should her verbal warning be ignored, she will administer a corrective nudge or nip to the hindquarters of the offending pup. These nips are not actually painful. They don't break the skin, and they are never delivered to the face, eyes, or fragile part of the pup's body. The pressure is only a hard enough to get the puppy's attention. However, the correction is delivered immediately while the offensive action is occurring. The mother's attention is already focused on her pup, and she is close by so that her lightning reflexes are fast enough to catch the pup in the act. She is not on the other side of the house, nor is she checking her social media news feed. She does not punish the pup after the fact. Furthermore, when the offensive action stops, so does the correction. She does not "ground" the pup by taking away all the toys for a week. This instant response is a form of "marking" because it occurs at almost exactly the same time as the behavior the mother dog wishes to correct.

Compared to how dogs do correction, humans do it badly. Most of the negative reinforcement we deliver is painful, scary, and well after the fact. That makes it completely ineffective, because the animal does not associate the punishment with the offense. Like the second girl in the dress code story, most animals associate punishment with whatever is nearest in terms of time and place. If you rub a dog's nose in the urine puddle he or she left on a carpet, the dog associates the punishment with your disfavor and your presence. He or she might engage in appeasement behavior and act "guilty" but the behavior itself will often not change. Likewise, if you put a shock collar on a dog and zap him or her enough to get his or her attention, the dog may not associate the pain with the bad behavior. He or she may well associate it with the collar, or with you.

Using a remote control to provide a negative reinforcement or punishment, by the way, does fool a dog one bit. A dog is perfectly aware that you did something to make a TV come on, a buzzer ring, or a shock collar deliver its zap. Although dogs are not well versed in the physics and electronics behind wireless communication, they understand cause and effect. The dog is completely aware that you're controlling the distant device.

A negative marker has to be a word or sound that precedes something unpleasant, such as a treat being withdrawn or a game being ended. Once the dog associates the negative marker with your disapproval, which is not by itself a painful or bad thing, you can use a combination of positive markers (like clicks) and negative markers to reinforce behaviors that resemble what you want, or that bring the dog closer to what you intend.

Attention Recalls

An attention recall is similar to the call or recall you use when your dog is elsewhere and you want him or her to come to you. But instead of communicating with your dog across a distance (that is to say, using a recall command), you are asking the dog to overcome distraction.

An attention recall can be tactile, with a gentle touch or a specific twitch of the leash. My particular attention recall is a two-note whistle accompanied by a double touch of my index finger on the leash. It means: "stop what you're doing and pay attention to me". When Honeybits looks at me, I give her a click and a treat. This combination of behaviors rewards a dog who learns to maintain a low-grade level of attentiveness toward the handler regardless of what other distractions present themselves.

Physical Redirection

Sometimes, you just have to pick a puppy up and put him or her in time-out to settle down. If the dog is begging at the dinner table or will not leave house guests alone and has become agitated or highly aroused in the normal home environment, you must stop what you're doing and put the dog in a less challenging environment. If you do not, the animal remains fixated and engaged in a behavior that can become self-reinforcing or self-rewarding if it's allowed to continue.

Physical redirection has an equivalent in the animal world: the stoppage of play, for example, is one way dogs and wolves correct one another.

For a human, a correction might involve stopping a game of tug-of-war or a pretend battle if the puppy nips too hard. It might involve physically picking the dog up and holding him or her until a tantrum subsides. It might involve putting the dog in a quiet, dark, familiar, comfortable place for a few minutes, if the dog has been crate-trained to associate the place with safety. Or it might involve coming to a complete stop while on the daily walk if the dog doesn't respond to a command to walk nicely on the leash instead of pulling.

A dog who pulls at the leash to turn toward the park when *you* do not wish to walk that way will continue pulling as long as he or she thinks there's a chance that pulling will get him or her what he or she wants. If you pull back or jerk on the leash, that's an entirely separate behavior that, in the dog's mind, is not connected to his or her behavior. If you yank, yell, or punish, the dog's attention becomes focused on the punishment and his or her initial offense may well be forgotten only to be repeated later, possibly with extra anxiety next time you walk that way because the dog will remember where he or she was punished or dragged about. I like to deal with pulling by freezing in place. Freezing in place and letting the dog pull ineffectively for a moment will eventually allow the dog to conclude that pulling and straining at the leash *does not work*. The dog's attention eventually shifts away from whatever he or she was pulling at when the dog turns back to look at you and find out why you're not moving. At that point, you have an opportunity to signal to the dog to sit, lie down, or do something different.

Natural Consequences

An alternative to freezing in place, for a dog who is straining at the leash, is to abruptly relax the tension on the leash so that the dog lurches forward. This has to come as a surprise or else it's not effective. I don't necessarily *drop* the leash, but the sudden change of tension can get my dog's attention and cause her to stop straining and to look at me.

There was one memorable day down by the duck pond when Honeybits pulled on her leash and got a surprise she didn't like. It was the predictable natural consequence of pulling on her leash while on a steep, slippery slope with her nose only a couple inches above the water. She wouldn't listen to my attention recall and was fascinated with the green, murky surface and the waterfowl nearby. When I relaxed the leash, the Chihuahua actually face-planted in the water. She couldn't climb out—the bank was too steep—so she dog-paddled around for a while before I led her to a shallow spot where her little feet could reach the bottom. I kept hold of the leash and could have reeled her in like a carp if I'd wanted to at any time, so she was never in any actual danger. Nor was she actually afraid, because I'd been teaching her to swim in the bathtub since she was about six weeks old. It *was* hilarious to watch her figure a way out of the water while all the ducks, geese, and swans quacked their opinion of her dog paddling technique. Afterwards she shook herself off, tried to crawl into my shirt to dry off, and settled for sun-drying as we continued on our way through the park. She hasn't pulled toward the duck pond since. She walks along like a well-behaved little dog.

I suppose you could call the experience of falling nose-first into a stinky duck pond a form of negative reinforcement, but I ought to point out that it wasn't punishment. First, dogs don't think about stinky, slimy water the same way we do. For us, it's a gross-out. For a dog, it's playtime in a nice fragrant spa. The strategy of allowing my dog to fall in is something that worked for *my* dog, for two reasons. First, she is a strong swimmer so being in deep water was not terrifying for her. Second, being unable to climb out immediately when she wanted to was a mildly negative experience for her. So, the experience of falling in was negative enough for her to learn her lesson, but not so horrifying that it caused her to develop a fear of the water. For a dog big enough to jump back out, there would have been no negative component at all and so it could have worked as an accidental reward.

Generalization

Training needs to be repeated, in different places and contexts, until the dog begins to "generalize" the behavior. Instead of responding to the heel command or the sit command only at home or on the leash, the dog will eventually understand that the command is to be obeyed *at all times*. Likewise the dog will learn not only to point at the sound of a specific noise, but at all similar categories of noise such as sirens or alarms. By learning to get my attention through touch and then to lead me to something she thought I should know about—such as a kitchen fire in its early stages—Honeybits was able to take a general concept and apply it to a situation she had never seen before.

Like most dogs, Honeybits is not fond of fire. She also doesn't like strangers prowling around the house or approaching the tent when we're camping. But she's savvy enough to understand when she doesn't know what to do about something, and she's been taught how to get my attention without necessarily making noise or changing the situation. Overall, I think it's safe to say that my five-pound alert dog has literally saved my home from burning down along with alerting me to a home invasion burglary in progress. Both times, she showed sophisticated behavior modifications by doing something she had not been explicitly trained to do in the given context: she extrapolated her training to new situations and generalized categories of threats.

Chapter 11: Hostility

This chapter focuses on some of the challenges you may face when you are out in public with your dog. The hostility is not necessarily directed at you or your dog: it may be your own hostility. It's normal to experience anger when confronted with an unfair or irritating situation. But, sadly, you'll run into people who are hostile to you or to your dog.

People Who Dislike Dogs

There are people who are not fond of animals in general or of dogs in particular. They would prefer not to be around them under any circumstances. People who have had bad experiences with dogs are often fearful or anxious, especially if they were bitten as children. Dog allergies are real, and people who have severe allergic reactions are highly inconvenienced by service animals.

I've written elsewhere in this book about how one person's right to swing his or her fist ends where someone else's nose begins. For a person with dog allergies, it's difficult to be in an airplane or other space recently occupied by a service animal. We mitigate the problem to a point by making sure the animal doesn't climb into a chair, sit on the upholstery, or get into other people's space. But we can't do anything about dog dander.

There will always be people who don't like your dog simply because he or she exists. For this reason, the Public Access Test includes steps to ensure that your dog doesn't invade other people's personal space to solicit attention or to interact in any unwelcome way.

"Not everyone who sees you wants to pet you," I tell Honeybits from time to time. Since she's a naturally sociable little dog, and since she especially loves children, she didn't always understand why a person she wanted to play with would sometimes back away. As the puppy spaz wore off she learned better.

There are things you can do to minimize your service animal's impact on other people. Keeping the dog groomed and in the vest is important, and so is cleaning up after your dog. But behavior is the single most important aspect of your dog's public image. The mellower your dog is and the better he or she behaves, the less hostility you will experience from others.

Incidentally, people who ask you whether your animal is a service dog, and what tasks he or she is trained to perform, are *not* usually being hostile when they are employees, owners, or managers of a public space. They are well within their legal rights, and they have generally been trained to ask the question of *all* people who enter the park, building, or other establishment with animals.

People Who Think You're Getting Away with Something

Having a service dog, especially for a disability, is similar to having a parking placard that allows a person to use an accessible parking stall. It's visible evidence of a disability. However, because hearing loss is an invisible disability that isn't as externally obvious as an atrophied limb or signs of extreme old age, it won't be evident that you have a disability until you try to speak to someone. If you lost your hearing as an adult, you will still have a lot of the muscle memory that goes along with speech even if part of the natural feedback system is disrupted or missing. Not everyone can be helped with a cochlear implant or hearing aids: people with trauma or disease related hearing loss often lose specific frequency ranges while retaining others, so simply amplifying sound doesn't help. This means that, to a stranger, there's nothing to justify the presence of your service dog.

There are two kinds of people who will behave in a socially aggressive way once they decide you're getting away with something. Exactly what they do, and why they do it, depends on their basic attitude toward people with disabilities.

People Who Hate People with Disabilities

This section was hard for me to write. I threw out the first five drafts, because every time I tried to express my position or to present cogent arguments for it, my writing rapidly descended into polemic. Eventually I realized that the only way to write in a civilized fashion about people who hate me is to do my best to understand the emotional and mental world they occupy.

From time to time, toxic doctrines of the past gurgle out of the cesspool to which polite society has consigned them. Among the many odious notions making a resurgence today is the idea that people with disabilities don't deserve to take up space in the world, and that we represent a useless waste of resources that could better be devoted to making ordinary people elite or elite people even better. Although this idea was part of the culture in both Sparta and the pre-Columbian nation-state of Mictlán, it was more recently associated with Nazi-controlled Germany, where people with disabilities (along with a lot of other individuals) were rounded up and put to death so that their homes, possessions, and other resources could be redirected to people the government deemed more worthy. During the Nuremberg trials, when the full horror of the Nazi and Japanese "camps" and "scientific experiments" became known, most of humanity decided that we could do better and that helping people with disabilities become and remain fully contributing members of society was sound public policy. The fact that adaptive technology consumed money and resources was acceptable because it took large numbers of people off the welfare rolls by helping them support themselves at least partially. For a while, most people were willing to accept a minor inconvenience or expense to themselves in exchange for a public benefit from which they might not benefit.

I believe it is the rampant inequality in the United States and elsewhere that has put enough pressure on the middle and working classes to cause them to bitterly resent public spending. Large numbers of people have been working hard and doing everything "right" for decades, but they have nothing to show for it. They have taken on unprecedented amounts of student loans for education that does not pay for itself. But while their net worth remains stagnant or even falls over time, they watch wealth and income skyrocket for the elite. So, they feel ripped off. This phenomenon, which was brilliantly described in *The Broken Ladder* by Keith Payne, is a form of stress that has a quantitatively measurable effect on human health and lifespan.

Some people who are on the wrong side of an income or wealth inequality gap (or who feel or believe as though they are) develop feelings of resentment toward people they believe are receiving more help than they are. They bitterly resent anything that resembles a free ride or any form of assistance to others, because they are struggling financially with no hope in sight. Accordingly, many people are beginning to question whether wheelchair ramps, closed captioning, and other means intended to improve public access provided enough benefit to society to justify the inconvenience to themselves. Some are genuinely upset because accommodations for people with disabilities exist.

When you're out in public with your well-trained Hearing Ear dog, at least some of the people who see you will think about the time and money it took to train up a service animal for you, and think: *"That dog cost more than my car."* (They're right, by the way.) Exactly who paid for the dog's training doesn't matter: you've got something very nice, and in their minds it equates to several months' worth of take-home pay that they, themselves, could have put into something that would have changed the world. (More likely, they would have drank, smoked, or gambled it away because they have developed habits that are not conducive to personal excellence. But it is more fashionable to blame other people, so that's what they do.)

There are other phenomena that may explain the pervasive belief that people with disabilities are unworthy opportunists. Some people may have had a bad experience with a person who happened to have a disability. But far more people who feel threatened by people with disabilities happen to have a scarcity mentality. They believe life is a zero-sum game: if one person has more, it has to be at the expense of another person who has less. When such a person sees a "less worthy" person receiving resources, he or she often feels cheated or deprived. But the biggest sense of hurt comes when someone who by rights ought to be "beneath" them (due, for example, to a disability) manages to exceed them in some athletic, artistic, or intellectual pursuit.

A person with a scarcity mentality and a grudge against people with disabilities is quick to point out that if a blind person climbs Mount Everest or a man with one leg runs all the way across the North American continent, it is only possible because many other people provided support. True as that may be—we all benefit from education and infrastructure created by others, and we all stand metaphorically on the shoulders of giants—it does not necessarily follow that helping the disabled person results in less, or nothing, being available to the able. That's bad logic.

People who start out with a major disadvantage often accomplish extraordinary things because they receive help, resources, and instruction from experts or others who are willing to share. The cooperation comes not just from a desire to help a disadvantaged person but from a legitimate alignment of interests. People with a scarcity mentality can often exploit an alignment of interests that already exists, but they can seldom cause one to appear out of thin air. A person who *can* see a way to benefit others, despite having a disability himself or herself, can often create an alignment of interest wherein others become willing to share resources and knowledge. This idea, of course, is anathema to a "rugged individualist" type who is convinced he or she is solely responsible for his or her success, and that cooperating with others or receiving help is somehow a form of cheating.

The "self-made" crowd that manages to work its way up from modest beginnings contains people who genuinely don't believe that people with disabilities deserve help or resources from others. A former friend of mine, after a little bit too much wine, asserted that spending money or resources on people with disabilities was a waste compared to "investing" those resources in someone like herself. In her mind, she had never received anything from anybody. Yet, since I've known her for years, I was aware of a great deal of help she'd received from friends, charities, educational grants, and a low-rate preferred mortgage through a government system. Somehow, she was able to mentally edit all of that out and sell herself—and others—on the notion that nobody had ever supported her or helped her out. She ignored the fact that she herself had received lifesaving surgery on more than one occasion that she did not have to pay for entirely out of her own pocket, and that she had benefited from the help of others during her recovery. Never much of a reciprocator despite her other merits, she had no problem accepting help from other people, some of whom ironically did have disabilities. Yet she was furious at the idea that anybody should offer money or opportunities to a kid in a wheelchair to help him or her become a productive taxpayer or to simply enjoy a normal life. "No one paid for *me* to go to camp," she complained, ignoring the fact that people, including me, did indeed take her camping, hiking, fishing, and on vacation at our own expense even after she became an adult who (according to her own doctrine) should have been paying her own way.

To justify a "rugged individualist" self-narrative, people will rationalize all kinds of hatred toward others. It was surprising to find out that my close friend despises not just me, but a group that includes me. We're no longer close—obviously—but the depth of my former friend's contempt surprised me given the extent to which she'd benefited from my generosity and support in the past. She will not ridicule people with physical, emotional, and developmental disabilities in public, but she does it in private after a few drinks. The root cause of her hatred is that she believes she has been unfairly deprived of resources and opportunities, and she thinks that if the resources given to people with disabilities or a rough start in life had been directed to her instead she would have gone farther, achieved more, earned more, and—in her mind—contributed more to human society through taxes, resulting in a net gain for humanity.

A person with a sense of grievance, a scarcity mentality, and the idea that he or she is solely responsible for his or her own success, will often be hostile to anyone he or she perceives as receiving a benefit he or she does not also have. This includes the right to have a dog in an area where animals aren't allowed. He or she does not see an accommodation as a way to help you contribute to society, but as something that you unfairly get to enjoy at his or her expense.

Social Justice Warriors

Social justice warriors are people who have—or like to think they have—a positive attitude toward people with disabilities. They strongly support laws meant to accommodate and integrate people with disabilities. They consider themselves to be allies of the disabled community and many of them have a disability of their own. However, they believe they need to assertively or aggressively police people who don't "look" disabled or who don't match their definition of a disability. Since hearing loss is an invisible disability, be prepared for dirty looks, snide comments, or outright criticism from people who are either "more disabled than thou" or "allies of the community".

Social justice warriors are the same people who write snarky notes and leave them on the windshields of people with handicapped placards because they don't believe the placard holder deserves a handicapped parking stall. They are the same people who criticize others for using handicapped restroom stalls, or who photograph people using any handicapped facility so that they can post them on social media to shame that person for having a "fake" handicap. The people who behave this way aren't necessarily able-bodied: they sometimes have disabilities of their own but have also adopted a "more-disabled-than-thou" mentality.

The fact that many of the smear victims do in fact have invisible disabilities is not a blip on a social justice warrior's radar screen. Social justice warriors are obsessed with the notion that somebody, somewhere, doesn't deserve the benefits or accommodations they receive. They believe that persecuting people with invisible or non-obvious disabilities is a valuable public service. Since few social justice warriors have much in the way of physical courage, they mostly confine themselves to snarky comments intended to be overheard. Luckily, we're not physically capable of doing that. Most of the vitriol doesn't enter the world we occupy, simply because it is composed of mouth noise.

The verbal abuse and public confrontation created by social justice warriors only becomes a serious problem if the social justice warrior escalates to the point of physically interfering with you or with your dog. Generally social justice warriors confine themselves to verbal abuse, and most of their mouth noise stays outside the world we live in simply because we're not physically capable of picking it up since it's outside our line of sight.

Faking Service Dog Credentials is a Felony

If you happen to have a small, cute, portable Hearing Ear dog who doesn't fit the mainstream notion of a working animal, you will eventually face accusations from complete strangers who believe your dog isn't real and who have no problem criticizing or cross-examining you in public. Some of the questions come from people who are legitimately curious and who aren't aware that their interest in our medical problems is rude. Other questioners are more sinister: they want to expose you as a fake. The kind of person who does this is the same self-entitled jerk who takes it upon himself or herself to ridicule people who use handicapped placards despite not having a disability. Hearing loss, like any invisible disability, unfortunately makes you susceptible to this kind of interference. The fact that many people have preconceived notions of what a service dog should look like only enhances a jerk's instinct to meddle.

The sad fact is that people can and do pass pets off as service animals to take them to the mall or to other recreational locations. At times, poorly trained pets misbehave or even attack humans or other animals. This results in a bad reputation for service dogs and their handlers.

In nearly every state and country, it's illegal to pass an untrained animal off as a service dog. If you do so, you can be convicted of a felony offense. Depending on where you live, you may face a fine or even jail time. A felony conviction can also interfere with your job and promotion prospects: many employers refuse to hire felons regardless of the type of offense, and landlords have the right to refuse to rent to an applicant with a significant criminal record. Faking service dog credentials is not a violent crime like kidnapping or robbery, however it's in the same category as automobile theft. It's evidence not just of bad judgement but of extreme, *premeditated* bad judgement.

Think about all the things a person has to do to dress their animal up as a service dog. They have to deliberately seek out service dog attire and fake credentials. Such things are available online of course (we have to buy our gear somewhere!) Unfortunately, the companies that sell them don't verify that the people they're selling to have a legitimate use for them. A person who wishes to dress up a fake service dog must therefore do an Internet search, pick out the leash and vest, pick out an ID card from a company that supplies them, and make the purchase. They have to wait for the package to arrive, open the package, and put the gear on their dog. Then, they have to take their dog out into a place where pets are not allowed, such as a grocery store, using the gear to gain access. They have to lie to employees or business owners who ask the questions that are legally permissible ("Is that a service animal?" and "What tasks is this animal trained to perform?"). Finally, they have to allow their animal to behave egregiously enough for some arresting authority to be called. There are *layers* of dishonesty that must occur, and it's almost all premeditated. This is not a crime of opportunity, like the theft of a sports car left running with its keys in the ignition. Nor is it a crime of passion, like an argument that gets out of hand and leads to a physical fight in which one of the voluntary participants gets hurt. It's not even an accident or a misunderstanding.

As tempting as it would be to put the onus on service dog equipment companies to verify that their customers are buying their product for a legal purpose, I don't predict that it will happen in the near future. Companies that sell tactical police equipment such as bulletproof vests with trauma plates have easy access to a registry of law enforcement officers, who each have a unique badge number and employer. There's no corresponding national registry of service animals or their owners. Even if there were, and even if your national government put laws in place to establish such a registry and to require service dog equipment sellers to check the registry before every sale, many items are manufactured overseas where your laws do not apply.

There are legitimate arguments against requiring vendors to use a registry. There are perfectly legal reasons for a customer to want a service dog vest without needing or having a service dog. They might be making a movie or putting on a play that requires service dog gear as a prop. They might be educating the public about what a service animal looks like. They might be buying a gift for a family member or friend who owns a service animal, or as a donation to a charity that provides service animals for others. They might be professional dog trainers who need a supply of leashes and harnesses to train their customers who *do* have service animals. Therefore, any person can order and receive the same kind of equipment that legitimate service dogs use.

Beyond the felony punishments involving jail and fines, what really strikes fear into me is that a person caught with a fake service dog will receive the ultimate punishment: *they take your dog away*. While Honeybits was in training, I was terrified that I would accidentally say or do something that could be construed as "passing her off" as having completed her training when she had not yet done so. I therefore made sure not to misrepresent her status in any way. I was open about the fact that she was in training, and when we were turned away from a museum or other facility, I respected that decision. Losing Honeybits would be like losing what's left of my hearing, or my eyesight. Not only is she the love of my life and my reason for living, but I need the services that she provides.

Restaurant Hate

There are some environments that, dear as they are to the designers of the Public Access Test, are inherently difficult for service dogs and the people who have them. Restaurants are one such environment, and they are uniquely awful for people with hearing loss. I hate them with a passion, which is why they are in a chapter labeled "hostility".

Maybe you can relate.

First, there's the background noise that makes it impossible to carry on a conversation. The walls, ceiling, and floors are designed to reflect sound as much as possible so that everything sounds "hip" like people are having a good time. That's not an issue if you're profoundly Deaf, but not everybody is. If you're missing some frequencies but not others, or if you have some hearing, a chaotic and noisy background makes it even more difficult to pick out a conversation. Hearing aids aren't the answer. They amplify *all* sound in specific frequencies and the filtering technology isn't an exact science, the same software that filters out the speech of the person next to you (who is facing someone across the table) will amplify the bellow of the toddler five tables away simply because he's facing in your approximate direction.

There's a lot of background noise in a restaurant. There are speech and chewing noises from people at other tables. There's the shrieking of unattended brats, the clatter and smash of dishes in the kitchen, and the mandatory idiot box on the wall where the latest sportsball game is either in progress or being commented upon by people who constantly interrupt each other. Closed captioning is either disabled or several seconds behind and is grievously misspelled. Then there's the swishing and yodeling of the piped-in Muzak, where some surgically enhanced diva is tootling like a hamster on cocaine, begging for her dream lover to come rescue her. I'm limited to lip reading and to wondering who will come rescue *me* from this cacophonous slop house.

Very few restaurants have circular tables where people can actually see what everyone else is signing. For the most part, you're limited to signing to the people across the table from you. The same goes for lip reading. Unless you can see both of the other person's eyes, you're not in a good position to catch the thirty percent (or thereabouts) of the spoken language that *can* be lip-read. If the lights are fashionably dim it's difficult to do even that.

The food, in restaurants, is seldom designed to be eaten easily by a person with a disability. Nor is it particularly healthy. It's over-greased, over-salted, and balanced precariously in a tower so that any attempt to eat it results in a cascade of sauce into your lap. Everything is fried. It's fashionable to say it's "grilled" or "pan seared", but in reality the food is prepared in the fastest possible way unless there's something about it that can allow it to be held at serving temperature for hours at a time.

But the worst thing has to be the way we're treated.

I am not a fan of being treated like a second-class citizen when my money is as good as anyone else's. I don't like being baby-talked, patronized, or treated as a child. When a waitperson continues to call me "hon" or some other fake term of endearment after I ask her to stop, I'm tempted to bury a fork in her eye socket. I speak several languages, but baby talk isn't one of them. Sadly, if you politely ask to not be verbally degraded or insulted by the wait staff, most of them laugh off your objections or defend their right to continue using insulting language.

I don't think it's unreasonable to want to be treated with the same level of respect as other adults. If a male diner is "sir", then a female diner of the same age should be "ma'am", not "hon", "sweetheart", or "we". If a white customer is "sir" or "ma'am", then an African-American diner should not be "boy", "son", "girlfriend", or any of the other irritating nicknames. If an able-bodied person is "sir" or "ma'am", we should also be called "sir" or "ma'am" and treated with the same level of respect. Unfortunately, when it comes to the service industry derogatory speech and patronizing behavior is rampant.

There's something about a disability that inspires able-bodied people to talk down to us, but nowhere is it as blatant as in a restaurant (or perhaps the medical community). Wait staff don't see us as people, much less as customers who are worthy of respect because of our hard-won skills in calculus, circuit design, or whatever else generates a paycheck big enough for us to afford the restaurant meal plus a generous tip. I think that the root cause is most likely the fact that management, and some customers, have taught the wait staff to behave this way by treating them like disposable chattel. Sexual abuse is rampant in the restaurant industry. So is mandatory unpaid overtime and illegal tip "pools" that force staff to share their earnings with management. The minimum wage that is less than half the minimum wage earned by the person who washes the dishes most likely doesn't help, and neither does the obnoxious customer who makes unreasonable requests, treats the staff like garbage, and then tips badly. In such a toxic environment, I kind of understand how the nonsense rolls downhill.

The next odious part of restaurant activity involves unwanted touching. I don't like it when people touch my body without an invitation, but nowhere is it more of a problem than in a restaurant. Not only are people constantly brushing or squeezing by because there's not enough space to move between the tables, but wait staff tends to be handsy. I think it stems from the same kind of patronizing fake friendliness I described in the last two paragraphs. When a waiter won't stop touching my shoulder or forearm *after I ask him or her to stop*, I've got a strong impulse to amputate the offending limb with one of the poorly-washed steak knives, so that he or she learns to keep the other one to himself or herself.

Obviously it's not socially acceptable to maim people. Nor is it in good taste to dump uneaten soup over the head of every random stranger who interrupts my meal to ask inane, invasive questions that I've heard umpteen times before. Yet as you are probably aware, patronizing behavior is so universal if you go into a restaurant while visibly disabled—especially if you do so while being female, elderly, or a person of color—the odds are high that you will experience homicidal rage before the evening is out. Furthermore, you will be expected to tip the person who's inspiring it.

One of the only positive things about hearing loss is the fact that it's invisible. If necessary, we can remove our hearing aids and lip read our way through an evening at a restaurant and get by while passing as normal adults. If you enter the establishment with a service dog, suddenly your invisible disability will become visible, and you'll be at the mercy of the staff. Everything you say or do will be scrutinized and used to either support or refute a stereotype.

Given the choice between being publicly humiliated and being excluded, I actually prefer to be excluded. That way I can go somewhere else, have a good time, and pretend that idiots don't exist. But the opportunity to choose not to be patronized or manhandled is *before* entering the restaurant. I self-exclude almost daily and save a bundle of money in the process by entertaining friends and relatives at home. Once you walk or roll through the restaurant door, your choice disappears because someone else controls whether you're treated like a toddler or a sideshow freak. At a charity ball or a private home, at least you can eat and converse in an environment that isn't cacophonous and where you are treated like the welcome guest you are.

For reasons unexplained, large numbers of dog trainers think that restaurants are a place where people with disabilities actually want to be. That may be true for some, but it certainly isn't when it comes to hearing loss. Despite the fact that few hearing-impaired people voluntarily enter restaurants, they are considered an ideal place to teach a dog impulse control. Many interpretations of the Public Access Test require restaurant activity. This is just one more case of how people without impairments chronically fail to understand what our world is like and how our experience differs from theirs. It leads to the well-intentioned but mistaken belief that we want to waste our time and money pretending to be like them.

If restaurant behavior is part of the Public Access Test as administered by your trainer, you'll have to practice it with your dog. This is a significant lifestyle change for normal people for whom restaurant activity isn't a significant part of life. The practice involved will impose significant inconvenience and expense, especially if your dog is used to ignoring you during meals and wandering off somewhere else. A dog who has been a household pet will be harder to train for restaurant work, especially when a restaurant is such an unnatural and ridiculous place to be.

If you're upgrading your pet into a service animal, be prepared to make significant changes to your lifestyle to check off this particular box. Just keep telling yourself that you might stop in a restaurant at some point while you're traveling. Also, be grateful that the Public Access Test does not (yet) contain a casino, strip club, or whorehouse component.

Social Backlash

Backlash is a social phenomenon that occurs when large numbers of people feel as though they, personally, are being negatively affected by a social or legal change intended to benefit someone else. These feelings aren't always objectively reasonable. Sometimes people feel as though they lose status when someone else is elevated to the same level as themselves. Other times they resent having to subsidize other people by paying for something they don't use themselves. Others believe they are being treated unfairly by being held to a higher standard. Either way, they direct their resentment at the people they believe are responsible for imposing the inconvenience and unfairness on them.

Backlashes occurred after every major legal change intended to bring downtrodden people into a position of equality. Women's suffrage, anti-discrimination legislation, and landmark Supreme Court decisions such as Roe v. Wade and Obergefell have all produced backlashes. Some of them have taken the form of overt violence or deliberate and public attempts to force the government to legislate the inequality back in. Others are more subtle: snide remarks, deliberate attempts to not follow the law, or intentional attempts to make people who benefit from the legislation uncomfortable.

Sadly, the Americans with Disabilities Act has created a backlash. People who resent having to spend money on things that don't benefit them, or that don't benefit anyone they know, tend to also resent the ADA. The solution to the backlash against the ADA is to become friends with large numbers of people who ordinarily wouldn't meet or interact with someone with a disability. This means that each of us must sometimes step outside our comfort zone and have conversations with clueless strangers.

Most of the backlash against people with disabilities comes from people who don't have any themselves. A baby born in an upper-middle-class neighborhood has advantages that begin even before conception. Parents can afford effective birth control, so children are far more likely to be planned and wanted, and prenatal care is affordable. Furthermore, if a wealthy couple wants to end a pregnancy for any reason including medical problems, they can afford a discreet abortion no matter how draconian the local laws may be. Wealthy families have always been able to afford a "trip to Europe" for either an abortion or a baby given up for adoption. Thus, wealthy children are seldom born with severe disabilities that limit their physical or intellectual development, and they are seldom unwanted.

Once a baby is born to a wealthy family, he or she receives the best possible medical care plus concentrated resources and attention from adults. The child is shielded from harm to the extent possible, and is unlikely to be consistently bullied, left unsupervised in risky situations, abandoned, or abused. He or she is less likely than a poor child to experience hunger, malnutrition, preventable disease, accidents, or exposure to toxins. This means his or her odds of receiving a disabling injury are lower than average. Furthermore, he or she receives treatment for learning disabilities, autism, or other problems that cannot be diagnosed until after birth. A wealthy family has the luxury of a full-time caregiver: either one parent can stay home with the child, or they can afford live-in help. Those with surgically correctible medical problems such as strabismus, spinal curvature, or a club foot receive the surgery they need. If the child has problems in school, tutors are available to help the child absorb the material well enough to pass standardized tests.

After high school, the child can get by without performing serious manual labor. He or she need not take on difficult, dirty, or dangerous jobs to pay for college. Nor does he or she have to make a lot of money as an adult to live comfortably. The young adult therefore never has to set foot in a slaughterhouse, on a construction site, or on a rooftop. The back injuries, repetitive strain disorders, and joint dislocations that plague the working class simply don't happen to wealthy students.

After college or university the student from a wealthy family tends to land in the kind of job where they can continue to work despite a mild disability (such as hearing loss) and that does not expose them to the risk of being shot, blown up, electrocuted, or crushed by a falling tree. Should the young adult enter a military service, it is generally as an officer and not as an enlisted person. As an officer, the young adult is seldom exposed to serious physical risk. Given that injury and trauma is far more likely to occur to enlisted members than to officers, injuries related to military service are far more widespread among the poor.

With all the protection that wealth provides, and because people tend to be surrounded with others who are like themselves, many very privileged people are convinced that the wealth and comfort they accrue as adults is due solely to their own hard work and inherent merit. Not only is there a strong tendency to ignore the positive benefits of the very good start that an upper-middle-class or upper-class background provides, but there's a tendency to simply not believe that other people struggle. We just aren't part of the world they live in. So it's unreasonable to expect them to vote in favor of things that make it easier for us to get around in a world that wasn't designed for us. In their minds, "everyone" has access to live-in staff, private health insurance, home nursing care, an on-demand driver, and the money to pay for it all. They also have a very distorted idea about what insurance does or does not pay for, how low of a standard of living is required to qualify for medical assistance from the state, or the extent of the generational economic damage done to a family when someone has to rely on Medicaid.

People from wealthy backgrounds often truly believe that Medicaid is a gift of some sort. They do not realize that the parents, children, siblings, and grandchildren of a Medicaid recipient spend years contributing their own money to the upkeep of a sick relative. They postpone the purchase of a house and liquidate their own savings to take care of a beloved person. They forego education because they are busy providing in-home nursing care that is otherwise unaffordable or unavailable. The whole family sacrifices to keep Grandma or Grandpa in his or her own home. But then, after the Medicaid recipient dies, the government swoops in after the relative's death and gouges back every single cent from the estate. The result is that the family that spent years trying to keep an aging parent or grandparent in a comfortable location such as their own home end up losing every cent they contributed because all the assets are snatched away, including those they contributed. Thus two or even three generations end up set back or even impoverished by caring for just one person who is sick or disabled enough to need Medicaid. In the mind of a wealthy person, the fact that disabled elders or people from the working poor class can "get free medical care" translates to receiving the same standard of care that they themselves get, with no other cost or disruption to themselves or their families. It simply isn't true.

If you take your service dog out in public, especially into a place where pets aren't allowed, there will always be a few people who think you're *getting away with something*. "I wish I could take my dog everywhere," is something people have said to me frequently when I'm out in public with Honeybits or engaged in training. Some people act like it's a privilege to be alerted to an oncoming vehicle, a siren, or someone sneaking up behind them. They're already aware of these things, *because they can hear them*. They think that every day is a giant pet vacation, when in reality there's a time, effort, and logistics burden associated with bringing a four-footed medical device everywhere. We get used to it, but it's definitely not constant pet time. Nor have I ever felt that my disability is some kind of privilege. The loss of my professional music career, for example, and the need to make up my income in other ways, wasn't exactly a lark.

It's OK

You're not expected to be a saint. If you feel resentment or free-floating rage from time to time it's actually normal. It's OK to get tired of being polite, subtle, and accommodating. Being an "ambassador", such that people form an opinion of all hearing impaired people based on their interactions with you, is draining. It's reasonable to get tired of having to explain or justify your dog's presence to strangers. Unfortunately, if you respond sarcastically or in a short-tempered way, it reflects on the entire hearing impaired community. That simply goes with the territory when you're a minority.

I know I'm supposed to act as though simply being out in public or being allowed access to public areas is an immense privilege, instead of something I should take for granted like the able-bodied do. I know I'm supposed to behave as though someone's doing me a favor by admitting me into the public facilities my tax dollars help pay for. But I resent that expectation too.

If I were my dog, maybe I'd be excited about all the butt I'm expected to sniff. Dogs like that sort of thing. But I'm not a dog. So, the smell of all the butt I'm expected to kiss gets old after a while.

On the other hand, interacting with me is probably the best way to help able-bodied people understand the community I represent. So I try not to get so self-entitled or so self-absorbed that I become an even bigger jerk than I happen to be by accident. It's bad enough when my hearing loss causes misunderstandings or causes me to miss announcements or information that is obvious to everybody else. I don't have to compound the problem. So, I've decided to do my very best to ensure that Honeybits and I don't make other people's lives worse just by being present.

Insurance

As always, the health insurance company is the primary barrier between you and the medical care you need.

A service dog's training is not usually covered by health insurance. But insurance products are available to cover a dog's medical care. Some people even buy policies to insure the life of their service dog to help defer the expenses of training a new animal should the first one die prematurely. Insurance policies are not mandatory, but there are people who have them.

The fact that the acquisition of a service animal generally isn't covered by health insurance policies is, in my opinion, a positive thing. It means that health insurance companies do not interfere with the process of finding, training, and testing service animals. This is fantastic, because it removes a draconian middleman that not only inflates the price of medical care but that does its absolute best to ensure that customers stay sick and are denied access to necessary surgeries and treatment. Health insurance companies aren't there to help you get better or to help you adapt to a disability. They are there to make money, and the chief way in which they do that is to collect premiums while doing their absolute best to ensure you don't actually get access to products or services that can help you.

Since service dogs aren't medicine, and since they're not a kind of durable device that is covered by health insurance, the big unfriendly insurance company isn't going to interfere with your access to a dog.

There is no insurance based barrier to you getting the help you need, provided you do not expect them to pay for any aspect of it.

Most people, of course, don't have an income high enough to easily cover the cost of service dog training. There are charitable ventures that sometimes help if you belong to the specific group they serve, such as disabled veterans or people with a particular illness or disability.

Chapter 12: Where to Learn More

I've cited a few books that helped me better learn and understand how to train my service dog. They are not a substitute for help from a professional trainer but they will help provide a context for the information your trainer provides. They will also help you work with your dog at home.

Dog Psychology and Physiology

For a good introduction into dog psychology and physiology, check out the best-selling work *Inside of a Dog*, by Alexandra Horowitz. She provides information about everything from how a dog experiences color to the nonverbal signals they use to communicate with one another. This information is good because it will help you select materials for targeting that are more readily visible and identifiable to your dog.

Dog Training

To better understand operant conditioning and "shaping", read *The Behavior of Organisms* by B. F. Skinner. It was published in 1938 but some of the principles are still valid. However, due to the enormous variations between dog breeds and individuals within each breed, the same strategy of reward or negative reinforcement will not be equally effective with each individual. Dogs, like humans, are complex enough organisms to interpret the general rules and rationales behind behavioral reinforcement differently.

To understand clicker based training and the positive reinforcement concept, read Karen Pryor's *Don't Shoot the Dog*. Pryor's work is more practical than laboratory based, and she emphasizes positive reinforcement training instead of negative reinforcement. Pryor is particularly opposed to the use of necessary food as a reward for animals who are deliberately kept underweight or in semi-starvation conditions.

Cesar Millan is one of the most prolific and famous authors on the subject of dog training. My early reading consisted mostly of his essays, however I see that his discussion on dominance and "being the pack leader" is misconstrued by many people who interpret it as permission to bully their animals and to use force or negative reinforcement in a way that does not benefit the animal. However, Mr. Milan's insights about how to construct an early environment for a puppy that is conducive to learning and to good behavior are outstanding. In *How to Raise the Perfect Dog: Through Puppyhood and Beyond*, Cesar Millan and Melissa Joe Peltier describe in detail how to help dogs develop desirable behaviors by controlling their environments until the "good" behaviors become habitual.

Works Cited

Grogan, John. *Marley & Me: Life and Love with the World's Worst Dog.* Harper Collins, 2005.

Horowitz, Alexandra. *Inside Of A Dog: What Dogs See, Smell, and Know.* Scribner, 2010.

Milan, Cesar. Peltier, Melissa Jo. *How to Raise the Perfect Dog: Through Puppyhood and Beyond.* Three Rivers Press, 2009.

Payne, Keith. *The Broken Ladder: How Inequality Affects the Way We Think, Live, and Die.* Penguin, 2018.

Pryor, Karen. *Don't Shoot the Dog! The New Art of Teaching and Training.* Ringpress *Books*, 3rd edition, 2006.

Williams, R.A. *Sustainable Non-Profit Management.* Smashwords, 2016

Other Books by This Author

Williams, R.A. *Sustainable Non-Profit Management*. Smashwords, 2016.

Williams, R.A. *7 Servants of the Toxic Emperor: Enabling Roles and How to Break Out of Them*. Smashwords, 2017.